What doctors, medical professionals, and patients are saying about

BEAT YOUR A-FIB: THE ESSENTIAL GUIDE TO FINDING YOUR CURE

"This book can help a patient regain a sense of control and be an 'informed consumer' of healthcare. ...An essential resource and should be required reading for everyone from patients, to families, and healthcare providers."

> Dr. Steven C. Hao, MD, FACC, FHRS
> California Pacific Medical Center
> San Francisco, California

"This is a terrific book."

> Dr. Hugh Calkins, MD, FHRS, CCDS
> Johns Hopkins University and Hospital
> Baltimore, Maryland

"A truly patient-centric view of the struggles when dealing with atrial fibrillation and deciding on an optimal treatment option. I think patients will find your book extremely helpful and informative, chock-full of advice to help them make their own decisions and be more educated. Congrats!"

> Dr. Peter Mofrad, MD
> Washington Heart Rhythm Associates
> Washington, D.C., USA

"...really excellent; I give it 5 stars."

> Dr. Robert Fishel, MD
> Florida Electrophysiology Associates
> West Palm Beach, Florida

"Reflects a decade long work-in-progress and is sure to serve as a valuable resource to anyone seeking to find a cure for his or her Atrial Fibrillation. Highly recommended reading for those with A-Fib and enlightening for their treating physicians as well!"

> Dr. Walter Kerwin, MD
> Cedars-Sinai Medical Center
> Los Angeles, California

"Congratulations on a great book. It is well written, balanced and contains detailed and yet simple descriptions of many aspects of A-Fib."

> Dr. Moussa Mansour. MD
> Mass. General Hospital & Harvard Medical School
> Boston, Massachusetts

"Incredible job on the book!"

Dr. Wilber Su, MD, FHRS
Heart Rhythm Specialists of Arizona
Phoenix, Arizona

"Very well done... a useful resource for patients."

Dr. Jeffrey Olgin, MD
Director, UCSF - Electrophysiology Service
San Francisco, California

"Provides valuable information about A-Fib in an easily understood format to help A-Fib patients make informed choices and successfully advocate for themselves."

Michele Straube, Patient A-Fib-free after 30 years
Salt Lake City, Utah, USA

"...masterful. You managed to combine an encyclopedic compilation of information with the simplicity of presentation that enhances the delivery of the information to the reader. This is not an easy thing to do, but you have been very, very successful at it."

Ira David Levin, A-Fib patient
Rome, Italy

"...a superb book! A fulfillment of your resolve to share the knowledge gleaned from your own battle for a successful cure more than a decade ago when PVI was experimental."

Warren Welsh, Patient, A-Fib free after 13 years
Melbourne, Australia

"... very impressed! I think it's great work, and very helpful for everybody with the damned A-Fib, whether fixed or still going on! Thank you, Steve for your great input in this field!"

Max Jussila, A-Fib free
Shanghai, China

"It's really interesting to read the 'editorial comments' at the end of the personal stories. I like the format to get the information across in a way that people would remember; i.e., '...Oh yeah, that one guy had...and this helped him... I should definitely check that out with my doctor'. I like the [eBook] options to easily choose what to read by simply clicking and easily 'travel' back and forth between topics."

Nancy Thompson, A-Fib Free since April 2009
Garner, NC, USA

More of what medical professionals and patients are saying about
BEAT YOUR A-FIB: THE ESSENTIAL GUIDE TO FINDING YOUR CURE

"Easy to read, and your explanations are complete. Too often informational medical books for patients talk down to them, this book talks to them."

> Muriel Corcoran,
> Executive Director Boston Atrial Fibrillation Symposium

"I would have given my eye teeth to have had your book as my guide when I was first diagnosed with A-Fib.... It took me years to have the understanding of the A-Fib picture that some could gain with a careful reading of your work."

> Bob Whitehurst, Patient, A-Fib free
> Palm Coast, Florida, USA

"If I had it 10 years ago, it would have saved me 8 years of hell."

> Roy Salmon, Patient, A-Fib free
> Adelaide, Australia

"I particularly enjoyed reading the Personal Stories portion of the book."

> Ed Webb, Patient, A-Fib free
> Fort Lauderdale, Florida, USA

"...an informative book I wish I'd had when I was suffering with the 'fib'...would be comforting to those suffering with A-Fib, for no other reason, than to know there are so many others in the same boat with them."

> Dave Hess, Patient, A-Fib Free
> Scranton, PA, USA

"... a great looking book that will offer new AF patients a collection of great information on how to approach solving their problem."

> Ken Close, Patient , A-Fib free
> Loveland, OH, USA

"I wish I had had your book in May 2006 when I was first diagnosed and totally unaware. I am so thankful I found you at A-Fib.com in 2009 after three years in the dark."

> Rose Vernier, Patient, A-Fib Free
> Austin, Texas, USA

"... excellent resources for a wide range of individuals and their families. It can help newly diagnosed patients deal with the anxiety and fear of the "unknown", as well as shorten the amount of time and energy needed to research and select the best treatment options."

> Mark, Patient
> York Beach, Maine, USA

What A-Fib Steals from You

By Joan Schneider
A-Fib free after 10 years

❖

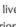

"I lived and put up with A-Fib for so long prior to my procedure. I had not realized just how much it had stolen from me.

Everything revolved around an episode... 'When was one due? Has it been a day since the last episode? Do I have any drugs in my pocket? I'd better schedule that appointment earlier in the day... most episodes occurred later in the day!'

It has been six months since my last episode, and I'm drug free! My quality of life has been restored after ten long years!

> *"I had not realized just how much it [A-Fib] had stolen from me."*

Just a few things I can now do without going into an episode: Hysterically laugh, sneeze, sleep on any side or position besides [just on] my right side, work a 16-hour day, watch a movie at a theater with loud bass, ride a roller coaster, exercise, wear out my 20-year-old children hiking in the Grand Canyon, go from 0 to 80 mph in four seconds in my Corvette....

Not to mention the 15 lbs. lost due to discontinuing the drugs (CVS Pharmacy misses me too!) I have three times the energy that has been missing for the last five years!

I cannot express how great it is to have my life back!"

Joan Schneider
Ann Arbor, MI, USA
A-Fib free after PVI catheter ablation

Beat Your A-Fib

The Essential Guide to Finding Your Cure

❖

Steve S. Ryan, PhD

WITH PATTI J. RYAN

❖

A-FIB, INC. ❖ MALIBU, CA

2012

A-Fib, Inc.
30765 Pacific Coast Hwy. Ste. 259
Malibu, CA 90265
Toll Free: 855-457-7146
DrSteveRyan@BeatYourA-Fib.com
PattiJRyan@BeatYourA-Fib.com

A Note to the Reader

This manual is intended to give general guidance on how to find appropriate treatments for your Atrial Fibrillation. The authors are not medical doctors and are not affiliated with any medical school, medical device company, pharmaceutical company, or medical practice. This information is not intended nor implied to be a substitute for professional medical advice.

Always seek the advice of your physician or other qualified health professional prior to starting any new treatment or with any questions you may have regarding a medical condition. Nothing contained in this publication is intended to be for medical diagnosis or treatment.

All unattributed quotations are by the authors.

The Internet: To the best of our knowledge, all web site links and addresses (URLs) listed in this book are correct at the time of publication. With the Internet changing daily, please excuse any URL errors due to changes after publication.

ISBN-10: 0984951407
ISBN-13: 978-0-9849514-0-6
PCN: 2011962960
Printed in the United States of America

A-Fib, Inc. is a non-profit entity dedicated to patient education for those with Atrial Fibrillation.

Table of Contents

❖

BY Walter Kerwin, MD

Within the pages of *BEAT YOUR A-FIB*, Dr. Steve Ryan, PhD, provides a comprehensive guide for persons seeking to find a cure for their Atrial Fibrillation, the most common heart rhythm disturbance in men and women. A-Fib, as it is commonly referred to, is both a disruptive heart rhythm and one associated with a lifetime increased risk of stroke.

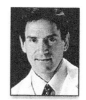

Dr. Walter Kerwin, MD
Cedars-Sinai Medical

Written in simple and easy-to-understand language, Dr. Ryan guides the reader through the maze of medical terminology to a better understanding of what it is like to live with this condition, what are the potential causes and how to research treatment options. Dr. Ryan provides a unique perspective as a person previously afflicted with A-Fib who successfully researched available treatment options and achieved an effective 'cure' of his A-Fib, allowing him to return to his passion of competitive running.

Since his cure, now over a decade ago, Dr. Ryan has served as a liaison between the A-Fib patient community and the group of physicians treating the disorder, the Cardiac Electrophysiologists. His website, *Atrial Fibrillation: Resources for Patients* (www.A-Fib.com) has proven to be one of the most trafficked sites on the internet dealing with Atrial Fibrillation, providing unbiased reportage of treatment advances, research findings and patient-to-patient exchanges of individual experiences.

> ❖ *"Highly recommended reading for those with A-Fib and enlightening for their treating physicians as well!"*
>
> Walter Kerwin M.D.

His newly minted guide, *BEAT YOUR A-FIB*, reflects a decade-long work-in-progress and is sure to serve as a valuable resource to anyone seeking to find a cure for his or her Atrial Fibrillation. Highly recommended reading for those with A-Fib and enlightening for their treating physicians as well!

Walter Kerwin, MD
Cedars-Sinai Medical Center
Los Angeles, California, USA

❖

INTRODUCTION

BY Steven C. Hao, MD

Atrial fibrillation can be a very terrifying and symptomatic disease. It can start out of the blue without warning which only adds to the sense of loss of control.

Medical terminology is often very confusing, and medical professionals seem to speak another language. All of this adds layers of anxiety and concern on top of the disconcerting symptoms of an irregular, often rapid heart rhythm.

Dr. Steven Hao, MD
Calif. Pacific Med. Ctr.

Atrial fibrillation has plagued mankind for centuries. Early physicians would see patients with rapid irregular heartbeats and learned that if the patient chewed the leaves of a certain plant, foxglove, they would feel better. We would later learn that foxglove contained digoxin which would slow the heart rate in Atrial Fibrillation. Subsequent research demonstrated the associated risk of stroke with Atrial Fibrillation and the protective effects of aspirin, warfarin, and later dabigatran.

Other medicines were developed with limited effectiveness in suppressing the symptoms of Atrial Fibrillation. But physicians still had the unfortunate task of telling patients that they would have to live with this disorder for the rest of their lives.

In the late 1990s, a medical group in Bordeaux, France, demonstrated that Atrial Fibrillation can be more organized than previously thought and effectively treated with catheter ablation. These advances have not only led to more research and breakthroughs, but also added to the complexity of pathophysiology and treatments for doctors, patients and families.

In *BEAT YOUR A-FIB: THE ESSENTIAL GUIDE TO FINDING YOUR CURE,* Steve Ryan has taken this chronic disorder and distilled it into easy-to-understand parts.

This book can help patients and families understand what is happening when a patient is first diagnosed with Atrial Fibrillation, the complicating issues, and the options for therapy. In *BEAT YOUR A-FIB,* medical terminology is decoded, and lists of questions are provided to start a conversation with your healthcare provider.

> ❖ *"This book can help a patient regain a sense of control and be an 'informed consumer' of healthcare."*
>
> Steven C. Hao, M.D.

This book can help a patient regain a sense of control and be an "informed consumer" of healthcare. This guide is an essential resource and should be required reading for everyone from patients, to families and healthcare providers.

Steven C. Hao, MD, FACC, FHRS
California Pacific Medical Center
San Francisco, California, USA

❖

PREFACE

My Promise to You

There are around 600 million cases of Atrial Fibrillation worldwide.[1] Each year in the US, there are over 460,000[2] newly diagnosed cases. In 1997, I became one of those new cases.

Atrial Fibrillation—I don't remember if I had ever heard the phrase. Then I developed A-Fib and began a year-and-a-half journey in search of my cure.

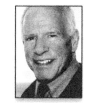

Steve S. Ryan, Ph.D.

Back then, the only information about A-Fib was written for medical students and physicians, i.e., professional journals, scholarly research and dissertations, scientific studies, pharmaceutical companies' and device manufacturers' "white papers", physician authored tomes, and medical school textbooks. Much of the advice about A-Fib was grossly outdated. And all of it was written in the language of doctors and medical researchers (and often still is today).

Despite my illness (and the associated depression), I spent months in medical school libraries. I studied the terminology of medicine and science. I learned to read and interpret scientific research, and to decipher my EKGs and operating room reports. I began speaking the language of my doctor. I conversed with top cardiologists and identified the current and best practices to treat (and cure) Atrial Fibrillation. I discovered cutting-edge techniques and where these procedures were being done.

> ❖ I studied the terminology of medicine and science... I began speaking the language of my doctor.
>
> STEVE S. RYAN, Ph.D.

I found my A-Fib cure in April 1998. But it had taken a lot of determination, courage, perspiration, and scholarly research. I vowed to share this knowledge with other patients suffering from A-Fib—to save them from what I went through to become free of Atrial Fibrillation. In 2002, I started my website, *Atrial Fibrillation: Resources for Patients* (A-Fib.com).

Flash forward to today. Thanks to this era of the internet and self-publishing, you have this book, **BEAT YOUR A-FIB: THE ESSENTIAL GUIDE TO FINDING YOUR CURE.** I've distilled everything I've learned about treating Atrial Fibrillation into one patient-centered resource written in plain language, not "medicalese"—saving you the time, depression, and frustration I went through searching for my cure.

My Promise to You: Through this book you will be empowered to seek and find your A-Fib cure just like I did.

In BEAT YOUR A-FIB, I offer you the information and insights to find your A-Fib cure. But finding your cure requires one more very important ingredient—courage. Courage—to seek another doctor if you're unhappy with your present one. Courage—to refuse to take a med you feel uncomfortable about. Courage—to seek the truth about A-Fib (sometimes despite prevailing opinions). And courage to select and pursue the best treatment option for you.

> MY PROMISE TO YOU
> ❖ *Through this book, you will be empowered to seek and find your A-Fib cure just like I did.*
> STEVE S. RYAN, PhD

You have that courage or you wouldn't be reading this book.

I dedicate this work to all the readers of A-Fib.com, to the hundreds of patients I have conversed with, and to the many medical professionals who have aided me in my quest. After more than ten years of continuing research, writing, and publishing a website designed for A-Fib patients, I'm thrilled to publish this patient guide in book form.

Steve S. Ryan, PHD
Malibu, California, USA

❖

"*My consultation with Steve Ryan was extremely helpful. I received excellent advice for my A-Fib condition along with names of reputable doctors to use for my treatment.*"

JOE REITMEYER, ELMHURST, IL, USA

"*Steve has the rare combination of in-depth knowledge and genuine kindness. He has been an invaluable and consistent support to me as I have navigated my way through various treatment options. I can wholeheartedly recommend him as an A-Fib coach; you will be most grateful to have him on your side.*"

KATHARINE, VANCOUVER B.C. CANADA

"*I have used the A-Fib Coach service on a number of occasions. It is extremely reassuring to have someone who knows the field inside-out take the time to really listen to you and then give helpful advice. It is also reassuring to have this service easily available.*"

DAVID HOLZMAN, LEXINGTON MA

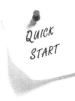

Your Quick Start Guide

In this section you'll learn about:

- Is this book for you?
- Why should you read this book?
- My journey to an A-Fib cure
- How to use this book
- Your 'free gift with purchase' bonus!

IS THIS BOOK FOR YOU?

Take our self-scoring quiz. No need to write anything down. Just ask yourself:

- Has your "quality of life" suffered because of A-Fib?
- Are you scared or frightened?
- Are you looking for impartial information—from someone not associated with a specific treatment, pharmaceutical company, HMO, or with your medical insurance provider?
- Do you need information written in plain language, not medical jargon?
- Do you want a cure and not just more medication?

If you answered "yes" to any of these questions, then BEAT YOUR A-FIB: THE ESSENTIAL GUIDE TO FINDING YOUR CURE is meant for you.

WHY SHOULD YOU READ THIS BOOK ANYWAY?

In 1998, I beat my A-Fib. Through extensive research in medical school libraries, by studying research journals, and by interviewing the leading specialists who treat A-Fib, I found my A-Fib cure. So can you.

In 2002, I started my website, *Atrial Fibrillation: Resources for Patients* (www.A-Fib.com). I poured everything I learned about my own cure into the website. But that was only the beginning. I broadened my knowledge of A-Fib beyond my own case, learning about new research and developments in the treatment of A-Fib. I continued corresponding with leading A-Fib specialists, and began many, many conversations with fellow A-Fib patients.

In 2003, I began attending the annual *Boston Atrial Fibrillation Symposium* where cardiologists, electrophysiologists and researchers present their findings and discuss cutting-edge treatments for A-Fib. I report these findings on A-Fib.com.

The good news: much has been learned in the last decade regarding the underlying mechanisms of A-Fib. This has led to improved treatments and procedures—offering many patients a life free of A-Fib.

The bad news: the number of A-Fib cases is growing yearly from the nearly 3 million in the United States now to an estimated figure over 16 million by the year 2050 (with similar trends worldwide). [3, 4]

I continue to study, question and learn about A-Fib. I've made it my mission to share this knowledge with others to help them become free of A-Fib.

My website content is continuously updated and expanded. Thousands visit my website every month. Hundreds of A-Fib patients write me every year about how to fix their A-Fib and are grateful for the information and advice I offer.

I've distilled all I've learned down to the essentials and presented it in an easy-to-read format. BEAT YOUR A-FIB: THE ESSENTIAL GUIDE TO FINDING YOUR CURE gives you unbiased information about A-Fib treatments, helps you choose the right doctor and/or medical center, and arms you to find your A-Fib cure. In addition, we hope to inspire you through the personal experiences and advice of those who have had A-Fib and been cured.

> ❖ *I've distilled all I've learned to the essentials and presented it in an easy-to-read format.*
>
> STEVE S. RYAN, Ph.D.

BEAT YOUR A-FIB: THE ESSENTIAL GUIDE TO FINDING YOUR CURE is written for you—the patient—from your point of view. As much as possible, we translate medical terms and research into everyday language. All the same, medical journals and other sources are marked with footnotes and listed at the end of the book for those who wish to refer to the source material.

However, you will be introduced to many new medical terms. These terms are listed in our Glossary of Medical Terms (*Appendix A*) each with a brief, easy-to-understand definition.

MY JOURNEY TO A CURE

To read my entire story about developing A-Fib, disappointments with medications, multiple failed ablations, and my ultimate journey to a cure, see Appendix C.

HOW TO USE THIS BOOK

If you are interested in a particular topic, by all means, jump right in and read that chapter. Use the Glossary when unsure of a medical reference or term.

Our recommendation: To become an informed patient and advocate for your own cure, start at the beginning of the book and work your way through to the conclusion.

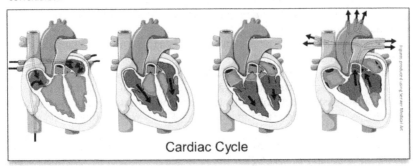

Cardiac Cycle

Visual 1: The Cardiac Cycle.

PART I is a medical review of A-Fib and its causes. Chapter 1 begins by describing what happens when your heart is in A-Fib. You'll learn about the associated risks of blot clots and stroke and the progressive nature of A-Fib causing damage to the heart, brain and other organs.

In Chapter 2, we answer the question, "How'd I get A-Fib?" by discussing the causes of Atrial Fibrillation. In Chapter 3, we'll answer the most Frequently Asked Questions (FAQs) about life with A-Fib.

PART II is all about treatments and procedures used to control or eliminate Atrial Fibrillation. Chapter 4 reviews the most common tests to diagnose or track your progress. Chapter 5 talks about the mineral deficiencies common with A-Fib patients. Chapter 6 covers medications (drug therapies) used in the treatment of A-Fib. Chapter 7 addresses the procedures and surgeries for treating and curing your A-Fib. Chapter 8 presents FAQs (Frequently Asked Questions) about A-Fib treatments.

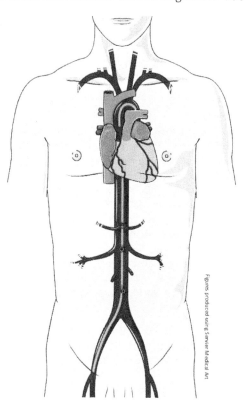

Visual 2: Veins leading to heart.

Figures produced using Servier Medical Art

PART III starts to map out your plan for finding your cure. In Chapter 9, we'll step through the most common patient scenarios and the treatment options recommended for each. In Chapter 10, we cover the types of physicians who treat A-Fib. We'll help you find the right doctor for you, including questions for "interviewing" doctors and how to interpret the answers they give you.

Chapter 11 shares stories of hope and courage from other A-Fib patients including first-hand advice. Following each patient story is a special feature, "Editorial Comments" with pertinent medical information and explanations to help you understand the problems or conditions described by the patient and offer insight as to their significance. And finally, in Chapter 12, we reveal the patients' "top ten list" of lessons learned, and offer steps to create your plan for finding your A-Fib cure.

PART IV contains our Appendices—full of useful information: an extensive Glossary of Medical Terms used in this book (Appendix A) and a slew of Recommended Resources and Website Links (Appendix B). In Appendix C, you can read my own A-Fib success story.

The **AFTERWORD** includes information about the authors, a special reader discount offer from the *A-Fib Coach*[SM], credits for all visuals used in the book, a Bibliography of all reference sources, the full web address for every web link and the list of Endnotes (references).

'PULL QUOTES' AND SIDEBARS

Throughout the book you will see 'call out' boxes or 'pull quotes' (like the example at right). These are designed to emphasize important information and perspectives, or to augment the content.

> ❖ "... emphasize important information & perspectives...."

In addition, photo sidebars (example at right) offer you a cross-reference to related content, i.e., relevant, first-hand patient experiences located in Chapter 11. It's up to you if you want to immediately "jump" to the story or just read it later.

REQUEST YOUR FREE GIFT WITH PURCHASE BONUS!

As a thank you gift for purchasing our book we want to offer you a FREE bonus: *"Questions for Doctors: Four Worksheets"*, a $9.99 value!

To receive your FREE gift, just send an email to FreeWorksheets@BeatYourA-Fib.com. We'll email you these handy forms in .PDF format; just save to your computer hard drive. The worksheets are based on lists of questions from Chapters 5 and 6.

Print copies of these worksheets and take them with you to your medical appointments. Use the worksheets to prompt important questions you should ask your doctor or medical service provider; each provides spaces for taking notes. Review the answers and your notes before making important decisions. File your worksheets with your personal medical records for future reference.

Ch.11: Personal Stories of Hope & Courage

Read how Jay and Kelly Teresi, and Max Jussila dealt with anxiety and stress.

SUMMARY

BEAT YOUR A-FIB introduces you to Atrial Fibrillation, its causes and the associated health risks. It gives you unbiased information about various A-Fib treatments, helps you choose the right doctor and/or medical center, and arms you to find your A-Fib cure. To encourage and inspire you, there are personal experiences of those who have had A-Fib and who offer their advice to help you find a future free of the burden of Atrial Fibrillation.

❖

Ready to start your journey to a life free of A-Fib? In Chapter 1 you'll learn about your heart in A-Fib, and the associated health risks if untreated.

❖

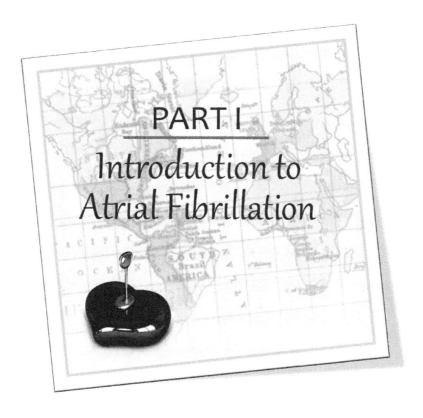

PART I

Introduction to Atrial Fibrillation

❖

"Never give up hope, and explore as widely as possible to find a way out.
… one needs to go beyond the doctors who advise patients to live with A-Fib."
Raju Tuladhar
Kathmandu, Nepal
(About her mother's successful ablation after 50 years of arrhythmia)

❖

CHAPTER ONE

Overview of Atrial Fibrillation

In this chapter you'll learn about:

- Parts of the heart
- Your heart in A-Fib
- Types and terms of A-Fib
- Atrial Flutter
- The health risks of A-Fib

You feel an uncomfortable flutter in your chest, or feel like your heart is going to jump out of your ribs, or that your heart is "flip-flopping around." Your pulse is irregular or more rapid than normal. You may feel lightheaded...very tired...short of breath...sweaty...and may have chest pain...

...and you may be a bit frightened and anxious.

Most patients with A-Fib experience one or more symptoms.[5]

Or perhaps you have few or no symptoms, and were surprised when the doctor said, "You have Atrial Fibrillation!"

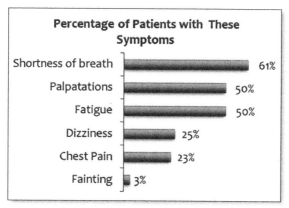

Visual 3 (chart): Percentage of patients with these symptoms
(patients could have multiple symptoms). [5]

YOUR HEART IN A-FIB

Sometimes the heart's electrical system may not work as it should and causes abnormal heart rhythms called arrhythmias.

When the heart is in arrhythmia, it may beat too quickly (tachycardia), too slowly (bradycardia), or in an irregular way. Atrial Fibrillation is a type of irregular heartbeat called supraventricular (above the ventricles) arrhythmia.

Hooked up to an Electrocardiogram (ECG or EKG), a normal beating heart, called Normal Sinus Rhythm, looks like this:

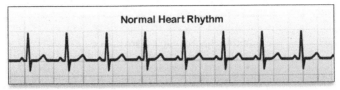

Visual 4: ECG strip of heart in normal sinus rhythm.

In A-Fib, the upper part of your heart is beating (quivering) faster than the rest of your heart. If you could look inside your chest, the top part of your heart would be shaking like JELL-O. One patient described their A-Fib as a "...motor idling too fast in my chest."

Somewhere in your heart extra electrical signals are being generated. This causes the top part of your heart to contract and quiver rapidly and irregularly (fibrillate) as many as 300–600 times a minute (the normal heart rate is 60–100 beats per minute).

In A-Fib, the ECG might look like this:

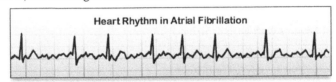

Visual 5: ECG strip of a heart in Atrial Fibrillation.

Notice the tracing shows tiny, irregular "fibrillation" waves between heartbeats; the rhythm is irregular and erratic.

PARTS OF THE HEART

Your heart is a muscular pump that beats close to 100,000 times a day. It's divided into four chambers—the left and right atrium located on the top and the two ventricles on the bottom.

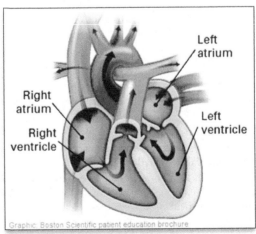

Visual 6: Heart ventricles and atria.

Normally each heartbeat starts in the right atrium where a specialized group of cells (the Sinus Node) generates an electrical signal that travels down a single electrical road (the AV Node) which connects the atria [plural of *atrium*] to the ventricles below. This electrical signal causes the heart to beat.

First, the atria contract pumping blood into the ventricles, then a fraction of a second later, the ventricles contract sending blood throughout the body. Normally the heart beats at 60–100 times per minute. (When a doctor or nurse takes your pulse, he/she is counting contractions of your ventricles.)

In the normal heart, the AV Node (in the right atrium) is the only electrical connection from the atria to the ventricles. But in A-Fib, electrical signals originate from other parts of the atria and disrupt your heart's normal rhythm. This causes the atria to beat or quiver on their own—sometimes as rapidly as 600 times a minute.

But only a small number of these atrial signals make it through the AV Node (which acts like a gatekeeper to the ventricles). This is fortunate, because you couldn't live with a heart beating that rapidly. The A-Fib signals that do make it through the AV Node make your whole heart beat irregularly and/or faster than normal.

TYPES OF A-FIB

A-Fib falls into general categories that describe the progression of the disease, ranging from occasional episodes to continuous or constant A-Fib. The categories describe the duration of your episodes, whether you experience symptoms and how severe they are, and whether or not your heart returns to normal beating (called normal sinus rhythm) on its own (spontaneously) or only with cardioversion (electrical or chemical shock).

In casual usage you may hear A-Fib described as occasional, persistent, and permanent or chronic A-Fib. Your doctor, however, may use one of the following medical terms:[6]

- **Paroxysmal:** (pronounced par-ok-SIZ-mal) describes episodes that stop on their own, and last anywhere from seconds or minutes, to hours or up to a week
- **Persistent:** episodes which last more than a week; or episodes lasting less than a week but only stopped by cardioversion
- **Long-standing Persistent:** a type of Persistent A-Fib that lasts longer than one year; (formerly called Chronic or Permanent)

Note: the terms Paroxysmal and Persistent are not mutually exclusive. You may have several episodes of paroxysmal A-Fib and occasional persistent A-Fib, or the reverse. Your A-Fib is called by whichever occurs most often.

A-Fib terminology can be intimidating (and confusing) at times. Some additional terms your doctor might use to describe your A-Fib include:

- **Silent A-Fib:** the patient feels no or very few symptoms; often discovered only during a routine medical exam.
- **Symptomatic A-Fib:** Atrial Fibrillation with noticeable symptoms (versus Asymptomatic or Silent A-Fib).

- **Lone A-Fib:** Atrial Fibrillation in younger patients (under 60 years old) in generally good health with no discernible cause or trigger (i.e., no other health-related problem or trauma); A-Fib is the "lone" health problem.
- **New** or **Recent-Onset A-Fib:** used to describe A-Fib during the 48–72 hours of first occurrence.
- **Vagal A-Fib:** occurs usually at night, after a meal, when resting after exercising, or when you have digestive problems; related to the Vagus nerve.
- **Adrenergic A-Fib:** occurs usually during the day and is normally triggered by exercise, stress, stimulants, exertion, etc.; related to adrenaline (epinephrine), a hormone and neurotransmitter.
- **Post-Operative A-Fib:** Atrial Fibrillation which arises during or soon after cardiac surgery; generally, it stops by itself. But sometimes the patient may require treatment.

WHAT IS ATRIAL FLUTTER? HOW IS IT DIFFERENT FROM A-FIB?

Atrial Flutter is another type of supraventricular arrhythmia. Some people have Atrial Flutter along with their A-Fib, or sometimes by itself without A-Fib.

In Atrial Flutter, the atria fibrillate in a coordinated, regular rhythm (for example, 300 beats per minute) rather than in a chaotic and disorganized manner as in A-Fib. (Like A-Fib, Flutter is an "electrical" problem of the heart versus a "plumbing" problem).

Consider Atrial Flutter as a more regular, milder variety of A-Fib. When Flutter occurs along with A-Fib, it frequently happens at the end of an A-Fib episode. Atrial Flutter often, though not always, originates in the right atrium, whereas A-Fib usually comes from the left atrium.

The following ECG strip (Visual 7) illustrates typical flutter in the right atrium with its distinct saw-tooth pattern. The "flutter waves" are noticeable throughout the ECG and are very easy to see in the rhythm strip.

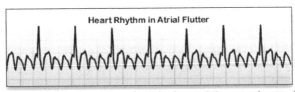

Heart Rhythm in Atrial Flutter

Visual 7: ECG strip of Atrial Flutter (with the characteristic saw-tooth pattern).

Right Atrial Flutter is easily cured with catheter ablation which can be considered a "first-line therapy" (typical initial treatment). *Note:* Flutter which appears *after* a Pulmonary Vein Isolation typically does not come from the right atrium and is harder to ablate.

HOW SERIOUS AN ILLNESS IS A-FIB?

A-Fib is the most common cardiac arrhythmia seen by doctors today.[7] A-Fib may feel weird and can be very frightening, but an attack of A-Fib by itself usually isn't life threatening.[8]

The biggest danger for those with A-Fib is from stroke (which is unrelated to your specific type of A-Fib.)[9] Blood clots can form and travel to the brain causing stroke. Because your atria aren't emptying out properly into the ventricles, blood can pool in your atria, particularly in the Left Atrial Appendage where most A-Fib clots originate. If a clot (thrombus) forms in the left atrium of the heart, it can dislodge and travel to an artery in the brain, blocking blood flow through the artery. The lack of blood flow to the portion of the brain fed by the artery causes a stroke.

If you have A-Fib and aren't being treated by a doctor, you are five-to-seven times more likely to have a stroke than the general population.[10] Researchers estimate that 35% of patients with A-Fib will suffer a stroke unless their A-Fib is treated.[11]

The American Heart Association states that A-Fib is a major cause of stroke, especially if you're older. It estimates that 15% of strokes come from untreated A-Fib.[12]

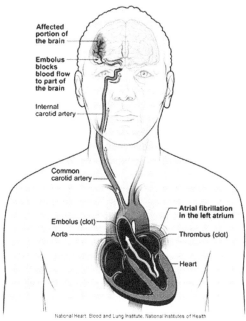

Visual 8: How a stroke can occur during Atrial Fibrillation.

Of those who suffered an A-Fib stroke, 25% had no prior diagnosis of A-Fib.[13, 14] Undiagnosed Atrial Fibrillation and a type called "Silent" A-Fib (i.e., with few or no symptoms), are very common. It's estimated that 30%–50% of people with A-Fib are unaware they have it (and the associated risk of stroke).[15, 16] (Everyone over 50 years old should routinely be tested for A-Fib as part of their normal yearly physical.)

And an A-Fib stroke is worse than other types of stroke. Half of all strokes associated with Atrial Fibrillation are major and disabling.[17] Of A-Fib stroke patients, 23% die and 44% suffer significant neurologic damage. This compares to only an 8% mortality rate from other causes of stroke.[18, 19]

There is also a danger of "silent A-Fib strokes" where stroke effects aren't evident but may appear like attention deficit, forgetfulness, and senile dementia.[20]

TALK TO YOUR DOCTOR ABOUT BLOOD THINNERS

The origin of 90%–95% of A-Fib-related strokes is the Left Atrial Appendage (LAA).[21] Blood flow may be slowed down in the LAA lobes and clots form when the heart's rhythm is interrupted by A-Fib. If you have A-Fib, your doctor will discuss blood thinners with you like aspirin, Plavix, warfarin (Coumadin), or dabigatran (Pradaxa) to help prevent blood clots from forming. (Aspirin is the lowest recommended, least effective level of blood thinner compared to Coumadin and Pradaxa.) Clots that can cause a stroke are an all-too-common happening for A-Fib patients.

Use of blood thinners is not a guarantee you will not have an A-Fib stroke. They reduce the risk of stroke by 60% to 70% in A-Fib patients[22], but that still leaves a significant chance of an A-Fib stroke. (The only 100% guarantee of not having an A-Fib stroke is to no longer have A-Fib—to find a cure for your A-Fib.)

However, if you are young, active, and have an otherwise normal heart, you and your doctor may decide your risk of A-Fib-related stroke is low, and you don't need a blood thinner at all.

Alternatives to Blood Thinners

But what if you need to be on blood thinners but are allergic to or intolerant of blood thinning medications, or you just don't want to be on blood thinners?

There are non-pharmaceutical options that can be used to trap blood clots before they exit the Left Atrial Appendage (LAA). The Atritech Watchman is an expandable device permanently implanted at the opening of the LAA. The Watchman is delivered using a catheter inserted into a vein through a small incision in your groin. (The Watchman is approved for use in Europe and is in clinical trials in the U.S.) [23, 24]

Another option is the FDA-approved SentreHeart Lariat II, a remote "noose-like" suture delivery system. Through a 4 mm incision made in the chest, a pre-tied suture is inserted from outside the heart to close off the LAA[25].

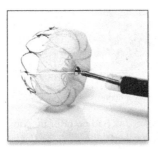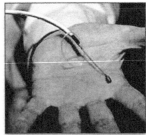

Visual 9: (L) the Watchman LAA Closure device from Atritech; (R) Lariat Remote Suture from SentreHeart.

With either procedure, closing off the LAA will somewhat decrease the amount of blood pumped by the heart. This may be of concern for people with physical lifestyles such as joggers, bicyclists, amateur and professional athletes.

A-FIB DAMAGES YOUR HEART, BRAIN AND OTHER ORGANS

If you have A-Fib, the upper parts of your heart (the atria) aren't pumping enough blood into the lower chambers of your heart (the ventricles). It's estimated this reduces the amount of blood flowing to the rest of your body by about 15%–30%.[26, 27] You may not be getting enough blood to your brain and other organs which may cause weakness, fatigue, dizziness, fainting spells, and shortness of breath.

Long-standing Persistent A-Fib has been found to significantly reduce blood flow to the brain and brain function.[28] Recent studies indicate that A-Fib reduces mental abilities,[29] and patients with A-Fib are 44% more likely to develop dementia.[30]

Inefficient atrial pumping puts an added burden on the ventricles. Prolonged A-Fib episodes may stretch and weaken the heart muscle.[31] Untreated A-Fib can also lead to more serious heart rhythm problems and to heart failure.[32] Of patients suffering from A-Fib, 20%–50% develop heart failure.[33]

PSYCHOLOGICAL AND EMOTIONAL EFFECTS

A-Fib can deeply affect your state of mind and emotional well-being. Research suggests that psychological distress is present in a substantial portion of A-Fib patients.[34]

The constant threat of an A-Fib attack, feelings of depression and impending doom, mood swings, and a sense of helplessness or lack of control are signs of distress experienced by many A-Fib patients. Anxiety appears to be the most dominant condition.[35]

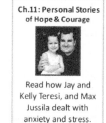

Ch.11: Personal Stories of Hope & Courage

Read how Jay and Kelly Teresi, and Max Jussila dealt with anxiety and stress.

A-Fib can have significant consequences on your social interactions, as well—with your family, friends and colleagues. Sometimes family and friends, and even your doctor, may not understand what you are going through—that A-Fib has a psychological component in addition to the physical.

Seek counseling and medical help when you experience any of these symptoms—your emotional well-being is just as important as your physical well-being.

A PROGRESSIVE DISEASE

It's important to treat your A-Fib as soon as practical. A-Fib begets A-Fib. If you have A-Fib long enough, your heart actually changes in a process called "remodeling." The fast, abnormal rhythm in your atria causes electrical changes and enlarges your atria. Your heart develops fibrosis, the formation of fibrous tissue in the heart. Your A-Fib episodes become more frequent and longer, often leading to continuous A-Fib. In a study of 5,000+ new A-Fib patients, 54% progressed to Long-standing Persistent A-Fib within one year.[36] However, some people never progress to more serious A-Fib stages.

❖ *It's important to treat your A-Fib as soon as practical. A-Fib begets A-Fib.*

This A-Fib remodeling holds true even for patients with no underlying health-related cause, called "Lone A-Fib." Over time, patients move out of the "Lone A-Fib" category due to aging and the development of cardiac abnormalities such as enlargement of the left atrium (remodeling of the heart). With these changes come the increased risks of stroke and death.[37]

But even with Persistent A-Fib, patients have been cured, and this remodeling of the heart partially or almost completely reversed.

So don't delay! The longer you wait to be treated, the worse your A-Fib could get. (If you've had A-Fib for six weeks, your A-Fib probably hasn't progressed very much. But if you've had A-Fib for six years, you should get treated as reasonably soon as possible.)

> ❖ *A-Fib is the most common cardiac arrhythmia seen by doctors today.*

SUMMARY

A-Fib is the most common cardiac arrhythmia seen by doctors today. An attack of A-Fib by itself usually isn't life threatening. The biggest danger from A-Fib is stroke. If you have A-Fib, it's most important to talk with your doctor about taking a blood thinner. Don't delay on this!

A-Fib can have both emotional and psychological effects, and impact your loved ones, as well.

It's important to treat your A-Fib as soon as practical. *A-Fib begets* A-Fib. Untreated A-Fib can also lead to more serious heart rhythm problems and to heart failure.

❖

Your next question may be, "How did I get A-Fib?" or "What causes A-Fib?"

In the next chapter we review the cardiac and non-cardiac conditions often associated with A-Fib, and other risk factors that can contribute to or trigger your Atrial Fibrillation.

❖

CHAPTER TWO
How Did I Get A-Fib?

In this chapter you'll learn about:

- Contributing health factors
- Cardiac conditions associated with A-Fib
- Other health conditions associated with A-Fib
- Lifestyle factors and other triggers

When your A-Fib is detected, your doctors will question you about your medical history, looking for contributing health factors. Do you have some other cardiovascular disease? Could another illness predispose you to A-Fib? Did the Atrial Fibrillation start after a surgical procedure, i.e., is it post-operative? Many times, though, A-Fib is seen in individuals without any overt heart disease.[38]

A-Fib is usually not something we cause or bring on ourselves. Often, there is no clear reason for one's A-Fib. Some events and diseases may make A-Fib more likely, but it can also occur without warning. When no specific cause can be identified, the following may be possible contributing risk factors.[39]

CARDIAC PROBLEMS

If you've had other heart problems, this could lead to diseased heart tissue which generates extra A-Fib pulses. Mitral Valve disease, Congestive Heart Failure, and Hypertension[40] (high blood pressure) seem to be related to A-Fib, possibly because they stretch and put pressure on the pulmonary veins where most A-Fib originates.

After open-heart surgery, up to 40% of heart patients develop A-Fib.[41] [42]

Ch.11: Personal Stories of Hope & Courage

Read how Ken Hungerford's A-Fib appeared after quad bypass surgery.

OTHER HEALTH PROBLEMS

Obesity,[43] diabetes, extreme fatigue, emotional stress, severe infections, severe pain and drug abuse can trigger A-Fib.

Low or high concentrations of minerals such as potassium, magnesium and calcium can trigger A-Fib.

Thyroid problems (hyperthyroidism), lung disease, reactive hypoglycemia and viral infections can trigger A-Fib.

Smoking cigarettes increases the risk of developing A-Fib even if one stops smoking, possibly because past smoking leaves behind permanent fibrotic damage to the atria which makes later A-Fib more likely.[44]

SLEEP APNEA

According to the National Sleep Foundation, sleep apnea affects more than 18 million Americans.[45] Instead of normal breathing, someone with sleep apnea has short or long pauses in breathing and/or shallow breathing occurring as many as 5 to 30 times an hour. About 4% of middle-aged men and 2% of middle-aged women have the condition. Sleep apnea is a much underdiagnosed disorder.[46, 47]

> ❖ *Many people have sleep apnea and don't know it.*

Research indicates sleep apnea may contribute to A-Fib, probably by causing stress to the Pulmonary Vein openings.[48] Many people have sleep apnea and don't know it. Your bed partner can tell you if you snore or your breathing repeatedly stops and starts as you sleep—often signs of sleep apnea. If you have A-Fib, it might be wise to have yourself checked for sleep apnea.

A Pulse Oximeter (about $50 in drug stores) can give you a "quick" analysis of how much oxygen is in your blood after awakening. A "normal" reading is in the 95%–100% range. A reading of 90%–95% would suggest that you're not getting enough oxygen when you sleep, that you need to have a sleep apnea study. (Below 90% indicates a bigger problem. You should see your doctor as soon as practical.)

AGING

A-Fib is associated with aging of the heart. As patients get older, the prevalence of A-Fib increases, roughly doubling with each decade. In the U.S., persons over 40 years old have an one-in-four lifetime risk of developing A-Fib.[49]

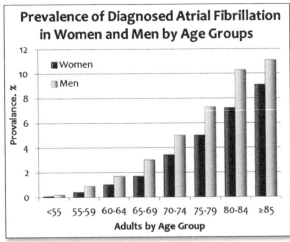

Visual 10 (chart): Prevalence of Atrial Fibrillation in Women and Men by Age Groups. [49]

Although A-Fib is rare in patients under 50, it is common among people in their 80s and 90s. In fact, 2%–3% of people in their 60s, 5%–6% of people in their 70s, and 8%–10% of people in their 80s have A-Fib.[50, 51, 52]

This suggests that A-Fib may be related to degenerative, age-related changes in the heart. Inflammation may contribute to the structural remodeling associated with A-Fib.[53]

Atrial fibrillation is uncommon in childhood except after cardiac surgery.

HEAVY ALCOHOL DRINKING

Heavy alcohol drinking may trigger A-Fib, what hospitals call "holiday heart." The majority of these A-Fib admissions occur over weekends or holidays when more alcohol is consumed.

Some researchers have detected no association between moderate alcohol use and A-Fib;[54] while others have found that moderate alcohol drinkers may have a greater risk of A-Fib than nondrinkers, though not as great as that for heavy drinkers.[55]

> Ch.11: Personal Stories
> of Hope & Courage
>
>
> Read about Kris and binge drinking.

GENETICS, PHYSICAL AND GENDER CHARACTERISTICS

Research indicates that an individual's risk of Atrial Fibrillation increases 40% if a first-degree relative (parent or sibling) has Atrial Fibrillation.[56] Genetics seem to play a larger role in younger A-Fib patients.[57] These findings are independent of research that has identified four rare genetic variants known to influence A-Fib risk.[58] (It's possible that people with A-Fib have a genetic predisposition not yet identified by current research.)[59]

> Ch.11: Personal Stories
> of Hope & Courage
>
>
> Read about Roger Meyer & three generations of A-Fib.

Athletes are more prone to A-Fib, perhaps because they have larger atria where there is more room for these extra electrical signals to develop and propagate, and possibly because of the extra pressure they put on their pulmonary veins through aerobic exercise.[60] Endurance athletes and other very fit individuals with low pulse rates are more prone to develop Vagal A-Fib.[61] A-Fib is often found in tall people particularly basketball players.[62] The risk increases markedly in 10 cm (4 inch) increments.[63]

❖...Overweight adults are 87% more likely to develop A-Fib.

Watch your weight. An article in The *American Heart Journal* cited studies that found overweight adults are 87% more likely to develop A-Fib than their normal-weight counterparts.[64]

Men are diagnosed more often than women, but women diagnosed with Atrial Fibrillation carry a longer-term risk of premature death. Atrial fibrillation is more likely associated with coronary artery disease in men, while Atrial Fibrillation is more likely associated with valve disease in women.[65] A-Fib is more common in whites than in blacks or Hispanics.[66]

A-FIB TRIGGERS

Some cases have been reported where antihistamines, bronchial inhalants, local anesthetics, medications such as sumatriptan (a headache drug),[67] MSG, cold beverages, high altitude, and even sleeping on one's left side or stomach are said to have triggered A-Fib. Antiarrhythmic meds to prevent or stop A-Fib can have a pro-arrhythmic effect is some patients.[68]

Heartburn (gastroesophageal reflux disease, or GERD)[69] and other stomach problems (like H. pylori) may be related to or trigger A-Fib.

Chocolate in large amounts may trigger attacks. Chocolate contains a little caffeine, but also contains the structurally related theobromine, a milder cardiac stimulant.

> ❖ Chocolate in large amounts may trigger attacks... The role of caffeine is debatable.

The role of caffeine is debatable. Research suggests that coffee and caffeine in moderate to heavy doses (2–3 cups to 10 cups/day) may <u>not</u> trigger or induce A-Fib.[70, 71, 72] Coffee (caffeine) may indeed counteract irregular heart rhythm.[73] But it's still a stimulant and may affect you and your A-Fib.

SUMMARY

A-Fib is usually not something we cause or bring on ourselves. Often, there is no clear reason for one's A-Fib. Some events and diseases may make A-Fib more likely, including other cardiovascular disease, other illnesses that predispose you to A-Fib, and after heart surgery. There are many risk factors or triggers that might contribute to A-Fib, but it can also occur without warning for no apparent reason.

❖

Did you identify any conditions or factors that may have contributed to your A-Fib or any A-Fib triggers that appear to be relevant to your A-Fib attacks? In our next chapter we will answer Frequently Asked Questions (FAQs) by newly diagnosed patients with Atrial Fibrillation.

❖

CHAPTER THREE

FAQs About Life with A-Fib

In this chapter you'll learn about life with A-Fib. Newly diagnosed A-Fib patients have many questions. In these Frequently Asked Questions (FAQs) and their answers, we hope to also address some of your concerns.

1. *Did I cause my Atrial Fibrillation? Am I responsible for getting A-Fib?*

    Most likely not. A-Fib is usually not something we cause or bring on ourselves. It's different from conditions like drug addiction.

2. *Is Atrial Fibrillation a prelude to a heart attack?*

    A-Fib is not a warning of an impending heart attack. A heart attack is a physical problem with your heart muscles or heart functions, for example, a blocked artery; whereas A-Fib is primarily an electrical or rhythm problem.

    However, untreated over a long period of time, A-Fib can eventually stretch and weaken your heart, and possibly lead to heart malfunction and a heart attack.

3. *Can I die from my Atrial Fibrillation?*

    Most episodes of A-Fib are not life threatening. It's not like having a heart attack.

    The biggest danger from A-Fib is the risk of stroke. Because your heart isn't pumping out properly, blood clots can form and travel to the brain causing a stroke.

    With A-Fib, you are five-to-seven times more likely to have a stroke than the general population.[9] It's important to discuss with your doctor if you need to take a blood thinner like warfarin (Coumadin), dabigatran (Pradaxa), or aspirin (less effective) to help prevent these clots from forming.

4. *My doctor says I have Atrial Fibrillation. Could it be something else? Should I get a second opinion?*

    A-Fib is fairly easy to diagnose using ECGs, Holter monitors, etc. If you have A-Fib symptoms and your cardiologist says you have A-Fib, you probably have A-Fib. A second opinion is more important when deciding *how to be treated* for your A-Fib.

5. *Will my A-Fib go away by itself?*

    Very rarely the cause of Paroxysmal (occasional) A-Fib does go away. In a process called "spontaneous remission" the body adjusts to whatever caused the A-Fib and the heart beats normally without any treatment at all. But don't count on this happening. You still need to be under a doctor's monitoring and care.

6. **Can I exercise if I have Atrial Fibrillation? How about my sex life?**

It's really a judgment call for you and your doctor whether or not you should exercise. If you can exercise without your heart rate becoming too rapid and you feel like exercising, you probably should. (In some types of A-Fib, moderate exercise may actually help you come out of an attack of A-Fib.).

The same applies to your sex life. You don't have to worry about dying while making love. Episodes of A-Fib are normally not life threatening.

7. **Can I drive my car if I have Atrial Fibrillation?**

In general, yes. With most types of A-Fib you can drive safely. But, if your A-Fib episodes cause you to become dizzy, as soon as you feel the beginning of an episode of A-Fib, pull off to the side of the road and stop. Wait there until the episode passes. If this happens often or if your episodes of A-Fib last a long time, you may need to stop driving entirely.

8. **Since I have A-Fib and am taking a blood thinner, should I carry an emergency contact wallet card or wear a medical bracelet? What information should I put on it?**

According to a paramedic with 25 years of experience, emergency measures to stop bleeding such as compresses, tourniquets, etc. will be used whether or not the paramedic knows one has A-Fib and is taking a blood thinner like Coumadin. But in general it's a great help to emergency personnel if one carries a medical ID.

INFORMATION TO CARRY WITH YOU:

In his book, *The Patient's Guide to Heart Rhythm Problems,*[74] Dr. Todd Cohen recommends carrying a "portable medical information kit" with the following information:

1. Full name and date of birth
2. Medical conditions
3. Implantable devices and materials
4. Allergies
5. Medications (and dosages)
6. A copy of a recent ECG
7. Contact information (family, your doctor, and your Health Care Proxy agent)

Type up the information, print, and trim; add a copy of your most recent ECG, then fold to fit your wallet or purse. Add a label, "In Case of Emergency" (ICE). See Appendix B for an online tool to print a free custom medical ID wallet card. Also, emergency personnel often look at your cell phone which should include the above info and where in your wallet or purse to find the ICE.

ADD A HEALTH CARE PROXY (POWER OF ATTORNEY)

A Health Care Proxy lets you appoint an "agent," someone you trust (such as a spouse, adult child, friend or religious leader) to make health care decisions if you're unable to. (See Appendix B for a free online do-it-yourself template.) Include your Proxy Agent contact info in your

Portable Medical Information Kit. Give a copy of your Health Care Proxy to each of your doctors for your medical records.

If you wear a medical bracelet or dog tags, include "see wallet card" in the text.

9.   **Is there anything I can do to get out of an A-Fib episode?**

Some patients report palpitations in which the atrium beats early. Premature atrial contractions (PACs) often occur prior to an A-Fib episode. If this is true for you, you may want to talk with your doctor about getting a prescription for an antiarrhythmic drug you can take when you get these PACs (called a "Pill-in-the-Pocket" treatment.) They may stop or shorten an A-Fib attack.

From our many A-Fib.com patient readers come the following suggestions. Note: these ideas are anecdotal, not scientific. Please use discretion when trying any of these methods.

During an A-Fib attack you can try:
*   Epsom Salt bath for twenty minutes
*   mild exercise
*   lying down in a darkened room
*   cold compresses or ice packs to the back of the neck
*   putting one's head between one's knees
*   breathing down hard on one's diaphragm
*   Immersing your head in a bucket of ice water

10.   **Is there any way to predict when I'm going to have an A-Fib attack?**

Try keeping a log or diary of your A-Fib episodes for three to six months. Note the time of day, what you were doing, what you were eating or drinking, etc.

By studying your log you may find, for example, that your A-Fib episodes come mostly in the morning, at night, or after a meal (which may mean you have Vagal A-Fib). Or you may find your episodes are triggered by exercise or exertion, by stress, or by stimulants (which may mean you have Adrenergic A-Fib). Some people notice very regular intervals between A-Fib attacks.

Observing these patterns may help you reduce your episodes or their intensity by avoiding personal "triggers" or help you better cope with them when they do occur. Discuss your findings with your doctor.

SUMMARY

Through these common patient questions, you've learned that A-Fib is rarely life-threatening, and that you probably didn't do something to cause it. A-Fib is not a prelude to a heart attack, and seldom goes away on its own. In general, it's okay to have sex, exercise, and drive your car.

❖

In Part 2 we cover the various treatments and procedures for controlling and curing your A-Fib. We start in Chapter 4 with the tests most often used to diagnosis your illness.

❖

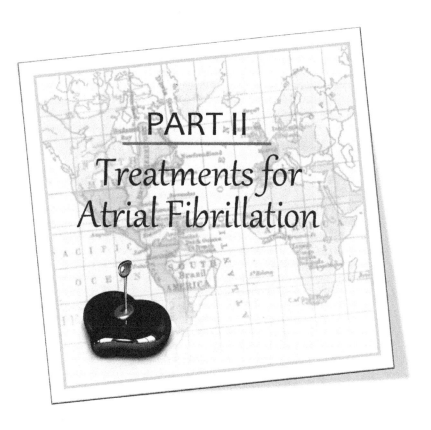

❖

"... My advice for someone with A-Fib is to thoroughly investigate
all your options and learn as much as you can."
Greg White
Free of A-Fib since 2008

❖

CHAPTER FOUR

Diagnostic Testing for A-Fib

In this chapter, you'll learn about the various diagnostic tests doctors use to identify and treat Atrial Fibrillation:

- Blood tests
- Electrocardiography (ECG or EKG)
- Holter and event monitors
- Stress test
- Tilt-table test
- Imaging technologies

There is no "typical" Atrial Fibrillation patient. Patients come for treatment at different times in their lives, and after having had A-Fib for different amounts of time. Doctors have several technologies and tests to aid them in evaluating your A-Fib. Your doctor will likely make use of several from this list.

BLOOD TESTS

Blood tests check the level of thyroid hormone, the balance of your body's electrolytes (i.e., potassium, magnesium, calcium, sodium, etc.), look for signs of infection, measure blood oxygen levels and hormone levels, and other possible indicators of an underlying cause of Atrial Fibrillation. Blood tests can also reveal whether a patient has anemia or problems with kidney function, which could complicate Atrial Fibrillation.

ELECTROCARDIOGRAPHY (ECG OR EKG)

An Electrocardiogram is a simple, painless test that uses up to twelve sensors attached to your body to create a graphical representation of the electrical activity of your heart. It won't detect an A-Fib episode unless it happens during the test. An Electrocardiogram is the most useful and often used test for diagnosing A-Fib.

The standard ECG records for only a few seconds. For a longer period of time, a portable ECG monitor is used. The two most common types of portable ECGs are Holter and event monitors.

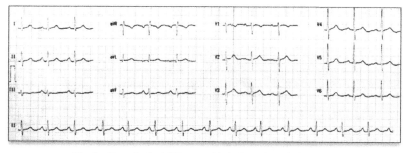

Visual 11: Normal 12 lead ECG trace with rhythm strip at the bottom.

HOLTER AND EVENT MONITORS

If you have occasional A-Fib (Paroxysmal), it's unlikely you will have an A-Fib episode while wired to an ECG in your doctor's office. So, doctors have other means of capturing your A-Fib data.

Holter Monitors

A Holter Monitor is a small, portable recorder that's clipped to a belt, kept in a pocket, or hung around your neck and worn during your normal daily activities. The leads from the Holter Monitor attach to your body like the sensors of an ECG.

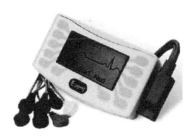

Visual 12: DigiCardio Holter monitor.

The Holter Monitor records your heart's electrical activity for a full 24–48 hour period in hopes of capturing data during an A-Fib attack.

Event Monitors

An Event Monitor is similar to a Holter Monitor, but it records data only when activated by the patient.

During an episode of A-Fib, pressing a button records several minutes of the A-Fib episode. (It's actually collecting data all along. When you press the button, it records several minutes preceding and several minutes afterward.)

Some Event Monitors start automatically when they sense abnormal heart rhythms. You might wear an event monitor for one to two months, or as long as it takes to get a recording of your heart during A-Fib.

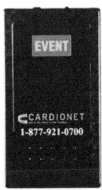

Visual 13: Cardionet chestplate Event Monitor: held directly to the chest to make recordings.

Implantable Monitors

A special type of event monitor is an Implantable Monitor. It's useful for patients with infrequent, unexplained fainting or passing-out when other tests have not found the cause.

Only a small incision is needed to insert the monitor under the skin (like a pacemaker), but it has no wires. The implantable monitor can be used for longer periods of time. It captures the length of A-Fib episodes.

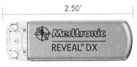

Visual 14: Medtronic Reveal® DX Implantable monitor.

EXERCISE STRESS TEST

Some heart problems are easier to diagnose when your heart is pushed to work hard. During a stress test, you walk (or jog) on a treadmill while an ECG records your heart's activity. This is often combined with an echocardiogram before and after the stress test to view and measure heart functions.

TILT-TABLE TEST

For patients who experience symptoms such as dizziness, fainting or light-headedness when neither the ECG nor the Holter reveal any arrhythmias, a tilt-table test may be performed.

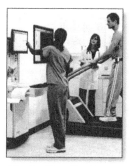

Visual 15: Stress Test System from CardiacScience.

The table tilts the patient upright at a 70–80 degree angle for 30–45 minutes. The test is used to monitor your blood pressure, heart rate and heart rhythm as you are moved from a horizontal to an upright position.

ELECTROPHYSIOLOGY STUDY

An electrophysiology study is a special catheterization test done to assess a patient's irregular heartbeats (arrhythmias) and is performed by an electrophysiologist (a specialist in the diagnosis and treatment of abnormal heart rhythms).

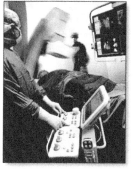

The electrophysiologist (EP) inserts several electrode catheters through the veins in your groin; then uses special real-time images, or moving X-rays (fluoroscopy) to guide the catheters into the heart.

Once the catheters are in place, the EP will use them to artificially stimulate or start your arrhythmia and record the electrical signals generated by the heart. (The doctor may also start and stop the arrhythmia using drugs.)

The catheters may be repositioned numerous times, and the pace of your heart altered through

Visual 16: Electrophysiology lab.

programmed stimulation. By recording and "pacing" from strategic locations within the heart, most kinds of cardiac arrhythmias can be fully documented.

This allows the electrophysiologist to examine the electrical activity inside your heart in order to determine if and why the rhythm is abnormal.

IMAGING TECHNOLOGIES

Echocardiography (Cardiac Ultrasound)

Echo uses ultrasound waves to create a moving picture of your heart. An ultrasound device is placed on your chest, and then special sound waves bounce off the structures of your heart. A computer converts them into pictures.

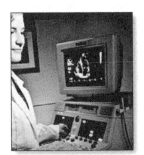

An Echocardiogram provides information about the size and shape of your heart and how well your heart chambers and valves are working. It can also identify areas of poor blood flow, areas of the heart that aren't contracting

Visual 17: Ultrasound equipment.

normally or are fibrillating, and previous injury to your heart muscle caused by poor blood flow. It's also useful in identifying and measuring any deformations of heart chambers and thickening of heart walls.

Transesophageal Echocardiography (TEE)

In this test, a tube with an ultrasound device is passed down through your esophagus in order to capture a clear image of the heart muscle and other parts of the heart.

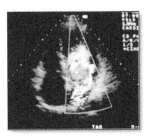

The ultrasound waves are directed into the heart, and the reflected sound waves picked up. A computer converts them into pictures.

Visual 18: Transesophageal Echocardiography.

The TEE is often administered just before an ablation to look for blood clots in your atria. If blood clots are found, anticoagulants are prescribed to dissolve them.

Computerized Tomography (CT) or Magnetic Resonance Imaging (MRI)

Cardiac CT uses an X-ray machine and a computer to take clear, detailed images of the heart and make a three-dimensional (3D) picture of your heart and chest to help an Electrophysiologist perform catheter ablations inside the heart.

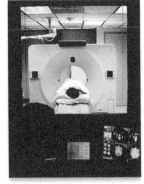

A cardiac MRI uses radio waves, magnets and a computer to create snapshots as well as videos of the beating heart. It can also be used to measure the amount of fibrosis in one's heart which can be a factor in the development of A-Fib.

Visual 19: CT Scan procedure rooms.

Chest X-ray

X-ray images help your doctor see the condition of your lungs and heart. A chest X-ray is a painless test that can show fluid buildup in the lungs, an enlarged heart, and other complications of A-Fib.

SUMMARY

There are several tests your doctor may use to evaluate your A-Fib. (You may have taken some of these tests already.) When your doctor requests or schedules any of these tests, your basic understanding of these tests helps you ask informed questions, talk over the appropriateness of specific tests and possible options, as well as discuss test results.

❖

Next, we will look at the minerals often deficient in the A-Fib patient. You will learn about the role some key minerals play in the healthy heart, and what to do if tests show you are deficient in these vital minerals.

❖

CHAPTER FIVE
Mineral Deficiencies

In this chapter you'll learn about:

- Testing for mineral imbalances or deficiencies common to A-Fib
- The importance of magnesium and potassium
- Warning about calcium levels
- Recommended formulas and dosages

An imbalance or deficiency in minerals like magnesium, potassium and calcium can force the heart into fatal arrhythmias.[75, 76] Your body's nerves and muscles depend upon these minerals, called electrolytes.

Magnesium is the fourth most abundant mineral in your body. It is important for coordinating the activity of the heart muscle and the nerves that initiate the heartbeat. If your magnesium levels are low, you are more likely to be at risk for arrhythmias (irregular heartbeats) and heart palpitations.

Potassium plays a vital role in the nervous system by ensuring that muscles contract properly. For the heart to produce a heartbeat, potassium must be present. Both high and low levels of potassium can cause irregular heart rhythms.

> ❖ *Unfortunately a great number of physicians...will dismiss your inquiries about nutritional supplements.*

There are many causes for an electrolyte imbalance such as loss of fluids (sweating, vomiting, chronic diarrhea, or high fever), use of antibiotics or diuretics, inadequate diet, malabsorption, stomach and hormonal disorders, or kidney disease. Replenishment is through food, drinks and supplements.

Unfortunately, a great number of physicians are not well versed in recommending or supervising nutritional support, and quite often may dismiss your inquiries about diet and nutritional supplements.[77] You may need to work with your doctor to determine the benefit of supplements for your A-Fib health.

TESTING FOR DEFICIENCIES

Before taking any supplements, have your doctor check your current mineral levels. Most will run a "blood serum test." But know that blood serum test results can be misleading. The body must keep serum levels within a tight range, or the heart stops. Consequently, serum levels are maintained at the expense of levels inside cells. Subsequently, essential minerals can appear normal in the blood and yet be deficient within the cell.

This is especially the case with minerals vital for heart health such as magnesium. For example, the body attempts to keep blood magnesium levels relatively stable and accomplishes this by releasing magnesium from bone and tissues. Therefore, levels of magnesium in the blood (an extracellular fluid) remain relatively stable (about 1%) even though working intracellular (within the cell) magnesium levels may be low.[78]

Nearly 99% of total body magnesium is in the bone or is intracellular.[79] Likewise, over 98% of body potassium is intracellular.[80] Measuring either using a blood sample is relatively insensitive, with small fluctuations in the blood corresponding to very large changes in the body's total reservoir.[81]

A more revealing test measures magnesium at the intracellular levels (such as the EXAtest[82]), but may not be readily available.

The red cell magnesium test (RBC) is another recommended option. Other methods for testing deficiencies of magnesium include the white blood cell magnesium test (WBC), the magnesium retention test (a 24-hour analysis of urine) and a sweat magnesium analysis monitored during an in-lab test.

Potassium levels can be tested with a red cell potassium test (RBC). [83, 84]

MAGNESIUM

"Anyone in A-Fib is almost certainly magnesium deficient."[85]

While magnesium (Mg) is one of the main components of heart cell functioning, it seems to be chronically lacking in most diets. "Magnesium deficiencies range from 50% to 68% in general populations in the US."[86] Most US adults ingest only about 270 mg of magnesium a day,[87] well below the modest magnesium recommended daily allowance

> ❖ *"Anyone in A-Fib is almost certainly Mg deficient."*

(RDA) for healthy adult males and females of 420 mg and 320 mg respectively.

This creates a substantial cumulative deficiency over months and years.

Magnesium Formulas

Magnesium supplements are used to build up your magnesium level. (*Note:* most multivitamins do not contain the needed supplement amount, although you may find some combined calcium-magnesium formulas that do.)[88] There are several magnesium supplements on the market in various forms.

Two forms of easily absorbed magnesium are:

- Magnesium glycinate: a chelated amino acid. Look for the label "Albion Minerals." This is a patented process designed to limit bowel sensitivity.[89]
- Angstrom magnesium[90]

Recommended Dosage (in addition to food sources)

In addition to the magnesium you consume through food, a recommended supplement dosage is a minimum 400 mg.[91] But higher dosages are recommended for those with risk factors for heart disease.

In the book, *The Magnesium Factor*, the authors suggest "you will probably need to build up your magnesium stores with more than 200 mg of extra magnesium per day. Supplement doses of 400-700 mg per day are common."[92] (Indeed, some researchers recommend a daily magnesium intake up to 1200 mg/day.)[93]

Supplemental doses should be spread throughout the day. For example, take 200 mg of magnesium two-three times during the day and another dose at bedtime.[94]

It's prudent to start off with very low doses of oral magnesium such as 100 mg. (Excess magnesium or magnesium sensitivity can cause loose stools and diarrhea which is counterproductive, because of the loss of electrolytes.) Increase the dosage of magnesium every 45 days. It may take as long as six months to replenish your intracellular magnesium levels.[95]

Your magnesium blood serum target is between 1.5–2.5 mEq/L (intracellular level between 33.9–41.9 mEq/L).

Alternatives to Oral Magnesium

If oral magnesium causes bowel sensitivity, an alternative (or an additional source of magnesium) is magnesium oil which is applied to the skin and over the heart.[96] A second method is to apply a drop the size of a quarter to the inner arm fold opposite and above the elbow, then wash off in 20 minutes.

Another treatment is an Epsom Salt bath. Soak for 20 minutes in a bath with 2 cups of Epsom Salt. (*Caution*: Epsom Salt baths can also cause loose stools.) You can also make an Epsom Salt spray—one part Epsom Salt to one part water. Place in a spray bottle and mist the chest. Let it dry on the skin.

DANGER OF TOO MUCH CALCIUM

Calcium (Ca) is essential for healthy bones, but it is also important for muscle contraction, heart action, nervous system maintenance, and normal blood clotting.

Leading electrophysiologist, Dr. Andrea Natale, warns that A-Fib patients may be consuming too much calcium. According to Dr. Natale, "calcium overload" is one of the primary factors in A-Fib's remodeling of the heart (i.e., changes in the size, shape, and function of the heart).[97]

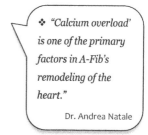

❖ *"Calcium overload' is one of the primary factors in A-Fib's remodeling of the heart."*

Dr. Andrea Natale

A-Fib patients may need to stop or lower significantly their calcium supplements, and increase magnesium. Magnesium works closely with calcium; calcium helps muscles contract and magnesium helps them relax. It is important to have an appropriate ratio of the two minerals in order for them to be effective.

Healthy adults usually need more calcium than magnesium (up to a ratio of two-to-one).[98] But for those with a magnesium deficiency, the ratio reverses. In the book, *The Magnesium Miracle*, Carol Dean, MD, ND, suggests those with definite magnesium deficiency symptoms take up to twice the amount of magnesium in ratio to calcium until their symptoms subside.[99]

Therefore, A-Fib patients should monitor their daily intake of calcium from both meals and supplements, and try to take in more magnesium than calcium (up to a two-to-one ratio).

The RDA of calcium for adults is 1000 mg (males)/1200 mg (females) with tolerable upper intake level of 2000 mg.[100] Normal calcium blood serum is in the range of 4.5–5.5 mEq/L (intracellular level between 3.2–5.0 mEq/L).

POTASSIUM

Potassium (K+) is often the second key deficiency for A-Fib patients. In fact, magnesium depletion can lead to potassium depletion.[101]

In the U.S., most women age 31 to 50 consume no more than half of the recommended amount of potassium, and men's intake is only moderately higher.

KEY ELECTROLYTES FOR HEART HEALTH	NORMAL BLOOD SERUM CONCENTRATION (Normal values may vary from laboratory to laboratory)	DESIRABLE INTRACELLULAR ELECTROLYTE CONCENTRATION
Magnesium	1.5–2.5 mEq/L	33.9–41.9 mEq/L
Calcium	4.5–5.5 mEq/L	3.2–5.0 mEq/L
Potassium	3.5–5.3 mEq/L	80.0–240.0 mEq/L

Visual 20 (table): Key electrolytes for heart health; Blood serum[102] & intracellular electrolyte concentrations[103,104] for magnesium, calcium and potassium.

Healthy adults should consume at least 4.7 grams (4700 mg) of potassium per day.[105]

Potassium helps prevent A-Fib by prolonging the refractory period—the time when the heart is resting between beats. (During this rest period the heart can't be stimulated to contract, thus leaving the heart in normal sinus rhythm.)

When potassium levels are too low, heart cells become unusually excitable, often leading to premature contractions and/or A-Fib.[106]

> ❖ *Potassium helps prevent A-Fib by prolonging the refractory period.*

Potassium Formula

There are several potassium supplements on the market, including potassium acetate, potassium bicarbonate, and potassium gluconate. (Potassium is sometimes paired with another mineral, such as with citric acid to make Potassium Citrate or with chloride for Potassium Chloride.)

Potassium supplements come is several forms including slow-release tablets and capsules, powder and liquid. The powder form of potassium—potassium gluconate (a chemical combination of potassium and glucose) —is easier to use than the pill form which is FDA–limited to 99 mg.

Recommended Dosage (in addition to food sources)

In addition to the potassium you consume through food, the recommended supplement dosage is 500-1000 mg[107] per day. This translates into 1–3 teaspoons of potassium gluconate powder[108] a day and should be taken with meals. As with magnesium, start off low, one teaspoon/day, and increase the dosage every four–five days.

You are aiming for a potassium blood serum level in the range of 3.5–5.3 mEq/L (intracellular range between 80.0–240.0 mEq/L). A word of caution—adding too much potassium too soon will make A-Fib worse, not better.[109] Too much potassium in blood plasma makes the cardiac cells depolarized and unexcitable, leading to spontaneous activity in other areas of the heart such as the pulmonary vein openings.[110]

KEY ELECTROLYTES	FOR HEALTHY ADULTS: RECOMMENDED DAILY MINIMUM OR INTAKE (FROM FOOD/WATER)	FOR A-FIB PATIENTS: RECOMMENDED DAILY SUPPLEMENT DOSAGE (FROM NON-FOOD SOURCES)
Magnesium	320 mg (females) 420 mg (males)	400-800 mg
Calcium	1200 mg (female) 1000 (males)	Mg > Ca (up to 2:1)
Potassium	4700 mg	500-1000 mg

Visual 21 (table): Recommended daily minimum or intake for healthy adults[111]; Recommended daily supplement dosage[112,113] of magnesium, calcium and potassium for A-Fib patients.

Alternative to Oral Potassium
Potassium gluconate powder can be added to bath water for additional absorption through the skin[114] (like Epsom Salt baths for absorbing magnesium).

OTHER NUTRITIONAL SUPPLEMENTS
You may want to discuss with your doctor other nutritional supplements often recommended for A-Fib, such as:
- Omega–3 Fish Oils
- Vitamin C
- Taurine
- Coenzyme Q10
- L-Carnitine
- Ribose (D-Ribose)
- Hawthorne Berry

QUESTIONS YOU SHOULD ASK
Most patients with A-Fib are deficient in magnesium and potassium and should monitor for an overload of calcium. Ask your doctor or healthcare professional:
1. What do my blood tests indicate about my mineral levels?
2. Do I have a deficiency in magnesium? A deficiency in potassium?
3. Could I be deficient at the intracellular level even if the blood serum test results are in the normal range?
4. Do I have an imbalance (overload) in calcium?
5. If I'm deficient in magnesium and/or potassium, can I take supplements to restore the proper levels?
6. Will supplements interfere with any of my other medications?
7. How often should I be re-tested for mineral deficiencies?

SUMMARY

An imbalance or deficiency in minerals like magnesium, potassium, and calcium can force the heart into fatal arrhythmias.[115, 116, 117]

Most patients with A-Fib are deficient in magnesium.[118] Magnesium depletion can lead to potassium depletion.[119]

Calcium overload should be avoided.[120] For a healthy heart, magnesium and potassium supplements may need to be taken over several months to restore the proper levels.

> ❖ An imbalance or deficiency in minerals...can force the heart into fatal arrhythmias.

Remember: Consult with your doctor before adding any minerals or supplements to your treatment plan. They may interfere or interact with the medications you are taking. In addition, you may need closer medical *supervision* while taking minerals and/or supplements.

❖

The next chapter covers the various categories of medicines prescribed for patients with A-Fib (known as Drug Therapies) and reviews the purpose and usefulness of each.

❖

CHAPTER SIX

Medicines (Drug Therapies)

In this chapter you'll learn about:

- Three drug therapy strategies
- The role of blood thinners
- Rate control vs. rhythm control
- Medications prescribed for A-Fib, and why
- What you can expect (or not) from drug therapy

When you have A-Fib, the strange medication names and medical jargon can be confusing and somewhat overwhelming. This chapter will give you a basic understanding of these meds so that you can be an intelligent participant in your own healing process.

The choice of medication depends on your type of Atrial Fibrillation, any underlying causes, your other medical conditions and other medications you take, as well as your overall health. For most patients with A-Fib, your doctor's first-line response (first choice of treatment) is usually drug therapy.

DRUG THERAPY STRATEGIES

There are three main ways medications are used to treat A-Fib (your doctor may use the phrase *Drug Therapy Strategies*). Drugs are used:

1. To prevent blood clots and stroke using blood thinners
2. To control the heart rate but leave the heart in A-Fib using rate control drugs
3. To stop the A-Fib and make your heart beat normally using rhythm control drugs

Drugs can be used one at a time (monotherapy) or in combination as a way to control heart rate during A-Fib, as a way to restore heart rhythm, or simply to reduce A-Fib symptoms.

BLOOD THINNERS

Your *absolute* first priority if you have A-Fib is to consult with your doctor about taking a blood thinner to reduce the risks of blood clots and stroke. Because the upper part of your heart isn't pumping out properly, blood clots can form and travel to your brain causing a stroke.

> ❖ *Blood clots can form and travel to your brain causing a stroke.*

Blood thinners don't actually thin the blood. Rather they inhibit the ability of substances in blood to form clots. They are more properly called "antithrombotic" or "anticlotting medications."

Clots are made up of two main components from the blood. These two components are *fibrin,* a long protein that binds together to form a mesh; and *platelets,* which are small cell particles that stick to the mesh and help to hold it together once they become active.

Drugs to stop the formation of *fibrin* are known as *anticoagulants*, while drugs that stop the activation of *platelets* are known as *antiplatelet* agents.

You may be prescribed an anticoagulant like warfarin (*Coumadin, Jantoven*) or dabigatran (Pradaxa)—a newly approved drug that acts as an anticoagulant. Some anticoagulants, like Lovenox and heparin, are given by injection (often used with hospitalized patients). Alternatively, you may be prescribed an antiplatelet like aspirin *(Ecotrin)*, *Ticlid*, or clopidogrel *(Plavix)*.

The anticoagulant warfarin (Coumadin) is by far the most prescribed blood thinner. In general, aspirin is less effective than warfarin.[121]

Warfarin Users: If taking warfarin (Coumadin), weekly tests may be needed to maintain the proper level, or you run the risk of a bleeding (hemorrhagic) or a clotting (ischemic) stroke. Even in the best clinical trials, only 70% of patients are able to keep warfarin within the desired therapeutic range.[122]

Good News: The newly approved drug, dabigatran (Pradaxa) is as effective as or better than warfarin and without many of the accompanying problems. Unlike warfarin, dabigatran does not require routine blood monitoring or related dose adjustments.[123]

> NOTE ABOUT DRUG NAMES
>
> We list the generic name of a medication first, and then follow with the brand name in parentheses. ❖

Dabigatran reaches an effective level within a few hours, which makes it simpler to schedule patients for a cardioversion or ablation; the drug can easily be stopped 24 hours before any elective surgery to prevent bleeding risks. For many patients dabigatran may replace warfarin as the blood thinner of choice for A-Fib.

> ❖ ...*blood thinners reduce but do not totally eliminate the risk of stroke.*

However, dabigatran is more expensive than warfarin, and patients taking it need to watch out for indigestion, burning, and stomach pain (leading to weight loss). As many as 35% of people taking Pradaxa may experience these symptoms (as compared to 24% of those taking warfarin).[124]

Caution: Blood thinners *reduce* but do not totally eliminate the risk of stroke.[125]

ALTERNATIVES TO BLOOD THINNERS

If you can't or don't want to take blood thinners, a non-pharmaceutical option can be used to trap blood clots before they exit the Left Atrial Appendage (LAA), where 90%–95% of A-Fib clots and strokes come from.

The Watchman is an expandable device permanently implanted at the opening of the LAA, and delivered via catheter (a long thin tube about the size of a piece of spaghetti) through a small incision in your groin. Use of the Atritech Watchman is approved in Europe but still in clinical trials in the U.S.[126, 127]

Another option is the FDA-approved SentreHeart Lariat II, a remote "noose-like" suture delivery system.

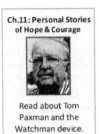

Ch.11: Personal Stories of Hope & Courage

Read about Tom Paxman and the Watchman device.

Through a 4 mm incision made in the chest, a pre-tied suture is inserted from outside the heart to close off the LAA.[128]

With either procedure, closing off the LAA will somewhat decrease the amount of blood pumped by the heart. This may be of concern for the young and for those with physical lifestyles such as joggers, bicyclists, amateur and professional athletes, etc.

RATE CONTROL MEDICATIONS

The next type of drug therapy, Rate Control, tries to control the heart rate (ventricular beats), but leaves the heart in A-Fib. This is an option when patients are relatively elderly, sedentary and with few symptoms (asymptomatic).

Medications used for rate control can be categorized as Calcium-channel blockers, Beta-blockers, and Cardiac Glycosides.

Left Atrial Appendage
Watchman device implanted via catheter

Visual 22: Left Atrial Appendage with catheter placing Watchman device.

Calcium-Channel Blockers

Calcium-channel blockers prevent or slow the flow of calcium into smooth muscle cells of the heart and blood vessels. Calcium-channel blockers are preferred (over other rate control choices) if you have heart or lung disease. Common side effects are: the heart beats too slowly, and constipation.[129]

Calcium-channel blockers include: diltiazem (Cardizem, Tilazem, and Cartia XT) and verapamil (Calan, Isoptin).

Beta-Blockers

Beta-blockers "block" the action of adrenaline. They slow down conduction through the heart and make the AV Node less sensitive to A-Fib impulses. Beta-blocker medications are better (than calcium-channel blockers) for active and/or young people. Common side effects are: the heart beats too slowly, tiredness and loss of sex-drive.[130]

Beta-blockers include atenolol (Tenormin), metoprolol (Lopressor, Toprol-XL), esmolol HCl (Brevibloc), propranolol (Inderal), timolol, pindolol, and the newer drugs carvedilol (Coreg) and nebivolol (Bystolic).

Good News: The newer drug, nebivolol (Bystolic), seems to eliminate some of the common unwanted side effects of beta blockers by dilating blood vessels through the release of nitric oxide.

Cardiac Glycosides

Cardiac Glycosides slow down and control the heart rate by blocking the electrical conduction between the atria and ventricles. The most widely prescribed Glycoside is digoxin (Lanoxin, Digitek), but medical authorities consider it the least effective rate control med.[131]

Be advised: If you are using any of the above rate control drugs, you probably will still have A-Fib. Only your lower heart (the ventricles) is controlled. You are still at risk of stroke and must continue taking blood thinners.[132]

❖ *Be advised: if you are using...rate control drugs, you probably will still have A-Fib.*

RHYTHM CONTROL MEDICATIONS
(ANTIARRHYTHMICS)

Another drug therapy treatment strategy uses rhythm control drugs, called antiarrhythmics, to try to *stop* the A-Fib and make your heart beat normally.[133] Rhythm control is usually the first treatment tried on A-Fib patients before proceeding to a catheter ablation.

Antiarrhythmics work by blocking specific chemical channels in the heart. "Rhythm control" means converting irregular rhythm to normal sinus rhythm and/or trying to prevent further episodes of A-Fib. This is usually the approach which is favored when the patient is relatively young, active and/or symptomatic from Atrial Fibrillation.

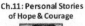

Ch.11: Personal Stories of Hope & Courage

Read about David Berkley's successful drug therapy.

Antiarrhythmic (anti-irregular heart rhythm) drugs fall into different drug classes (i.e., Class I–IV) because they work in different ways. Some classes and even certain drugs within a class are effective for particular rhythm disturbances.

These include:

- Class Ia (Sodium Channel Blocker) drugs include: procainamide, quinidine, and disopyramide (Norpace)
- Class Ic (Sodium Channel Blocker) drugs include flecainide and propafenone
- Class III (Potassium Channel Blocker) drugs include dofetilide, ibutilide, sotalol,[134] amiodarone[135] and dronedarone (Multaq)[136]

Ch.11: Personal Stories of Hope & Courage

Read about Kris and the side effects of amiodarone on her eyesight.

In general, antiarrhythmic drugs aren't very effective and tend to have unwanted side effects such as pulmonary fibrosis and impaired liver function.[137, 138, 139]

In particular, amiodarone, while effective for some A-Fib patients, has known toxic side effects particularly in the lungs, liver, thyroid and eyes.[140]

Antiarrhythmic drugs also become less effective over time, with approximately half of the patients eventually developing resistance to them. Up to 50% of patients experience a recurrence of A-Fib after one year of antiarrhythmic treatment, and up to 85% experience a recurrence after two years.[141]

Many antiarrhythmic drugs require you to be hospitalized initially for three–four days to monitor you for side effects. Because patients react differently to medications, some antiarrhythmic meds may sometimes promote cardiac arrhythmias (a pro-arrhythmic effect).

"Pill-in-the-Pocket" Treatment

The "Pill-in-the-Pocket" treatment refers to taking an antiarrhythmic med at the time of an A-Fib attack. (One objection to this treatment is that, like a brush fire, it's better to keep A-Fib from starting in the first place by taking antiarrhythmic meds on a regular basis, rather than trying to stop A-Fib after it starts. But not everyone can tolerate antiarrhythmic meds on a regular basis.)

A variation of the "Pill-in-the-Pocket" treatment is to take an antiarrhythmic med on a regular basis, then take a higher dose at the time of an A-Fib attack.

The Pill-in-the-Pocket treatment is *not* a "cure" for A-Fib, but is a stop-gap measure to get you out of an A-Fib attack.

QUESTIONS YOU SHOULD ASK

For most patients with A-Fib, your doctor's first-line response (first choice of treatment) is drug therapy. Before taking a prescription drug to treat your A-Fib, you should educate yourself about the drug(s).

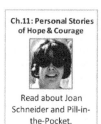

Ch.11: Personal Stories of Hope & Courage

Read about Joan Schneider and Pill-in-the-Pocket.

Ask your doctor or healthcare professional:

- Will this drug interfere with my other medications?
- How long before I know if this drug is working?
- How will I be monitored on this drug? How often?
- What are the side effects of this drug?
- What happens if this drug doesn't work?
- What if my A-Fib symptoms become worse?
- What if I don't respond to medications? Will you consider non-pharmaceutical treatments (such as a Pulmonary Vein Isolation procedure)?

SUMMARY

Remember: Your absolute first priority if you have A-Fib is to consult with your doctor about taking a blood thinner to reduce your risk of stroke.

As to *rate* control and *rhythm* control, don't expect miracles from drug therapies. The vast number of drugs currently available to treat A-Fib is an indication that none is wholly effective; each has limited usefulness, and is hindered by side effects and low tolerance by many patients.[142]

❖ *"Drugs don't cure A-Fib but merely keep it at bay."*

To date, the magic pill that will permanently cure your A-Fib probably doesn't exist.[143] "Drugs don't cure A-Fib but merely keep it at bay."[144]

So, let's move on to ways you and your doctor can fix your A-Fib (rather than just control the symptoms). In the next chapter we will cover the leading procedures and surgeries aimed at getting you free of A-Fib.

❖

CHAPTER SEVEN

Procedures and Surgeries

In this chapter you'll learn about non-drug procedures and surgical operations which aim to correct, treat or eliminate your A-Fib including:

- Chemical and electrical cardioversion
- Pulmonary Vein Isolation (PVI)
- AV Node Ablation with Pacemaker
- The Cox-Maze and Mini-Maze surgeries
- Pacemakers and Internal Cardioverter Defibrillators (ICDs)

The key to stopping your A-Fib is to eliminate the extra electrical pulses Atrial Fibrillation generates. Many factors influence the best choice of method for your A-Fib. The good news for people with Atrial Fibrillation is that there are a greater range of and more effective treatments than ever before.

CARDIOVERSION

The goal of cardioversion is to return an irregularly beating heart to its regular rhythm (normal sinus rhythm). This can be done with drugs and/or electrically.

Chemical Cardioversion

Chemical cardioversion is usually done in a hospital. A combination of meds is administered intravenously, such as Cardizem, verapamil, ibutilide, or adenosine. Doctors monitor you closely for adverse side effects such as nausea and fatigue, as well as for some long-term risks. Chemical cardioversion is often done in combination with Electrical Cardioversion.

Electrical Cardioversion

Sometimes an electrical shock can return your heartbeat to normal. During Electrical Cardioversion the patient is anesthetized and unconscious. A defibrillator is used (with paddles or patches) to shock the heart for a split second. The shock causes signal producing areas of your heart to discharge all at once. This stops all electrical activity in your heart momentarily, hopefully allowing your normal heart rhythm to take over.

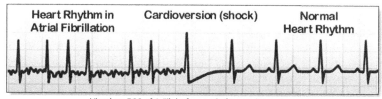

Visual 23: ECG of A-Fib before and after cardioversion.

Electrical Cardioversion, often combined with Chemical Cardioversion, is considered a standard, routine, low risk treatment option, particularly for patients who recently developed A-Fib. Electrical Cardioversion does have a high risk of forming clots and causing stroke[145], which is why it is important to be taking anticoagulants like warfarin (Coumadin) both before the treatment and in the three to four weeks following treatment.[146]

Electrical Cardioversion may successfully restore regular heart rhythm in more than 95 percent of patients. However, "50 to 75 percent of patients eventually develop Atrial Fibrillation again."[147]

Don't be frightened by cardioversion scenes in TV medical dramas. They may look and sound traumatic; but in reality, electrical cardioversion is non-invasive and is one of the easiest and safest short term treatments available for A-Fib.

PULMONARY VEIN ISOLATION (PVI)

Catheter-based ablation techniques are used to remove or disrupt the faulty electrical pathways in the heart that cause A-Fib.[148] Electrically destroying or "isolating" these signal areas keeps Atrial Fibrillation from occurring.

About 90% of A-Fib signals arise from the pulmonary vein (PV) openings located in the left atrium.[149] The pulmonary veins are large blood vessels that carry bright red, clean, oxygenated blood from the lungs to the left atrium. There are four pulmonary veins, two from each lung. The pulmonary veins most commonly associated with Atrial Fibrillation are the two upper veins (left and right).

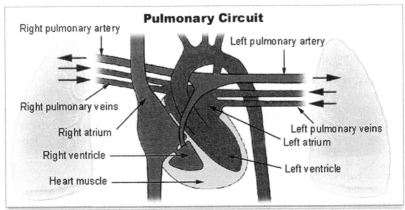

Visual 24: The Pulmonary Circuit.
Oxygen-rich blood flows into the heart; oxygen-depleted blood flows out.

Pulmonary Vein Isolation (PVI) catheter ablation is a non-surgical procedure performed in an electrophysiology laboratory. A PVI catheter ablation is a low-risk procedure, comparable to other routine procedures such as a tubal ligation.[150]

The Pulmonary Vein Isolation Procedure

Before the ablation begins, an imaging system such as a CT or MRI makes real-time moving images of your heart. This information is imported to special 3–D mapping equipment to create an electrical "road map" of your heart.

During the ablation a soft, thin, flexible tube (catheter) with an electrode at the tip is inserted through a vein in your groin, your wrist and/or neck. The catheter is about the diameter of the lead in a normal pencil, while your vein is close to the diameter of your pinky finger.[151]

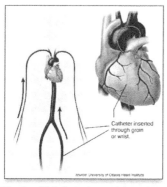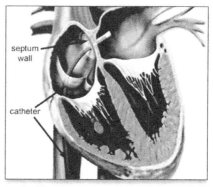

Visual 25: (L) Catheter inserted through groin or wrist; (R) Catheter advanced through septum (wall) into left atrium.

Using continuous "live" images created by a fluoroscope (a special type of X-ray), the catheter is moved up into the right atrium of your heart; then the septum (wall) between the right and left atria is punctured.

The catheter is then advanced through the septum into the left atrium and navigated to the Pulmonary Vein openings. The tip of the ablation catheter then delivers energy which burns or "ablates" a tiny spot of tissue, or "isolates" it. This process is repeated for each location. Most healthy heart tissue is left unharmed.

Frequently, other areas besides the Pulmonary Veins are involved in triggering or maintaining Atrial Fibrillation. They are also targeted and "isolated."

These ablation scars prevent the abnormal signals that cause Atrial Fibrillation from reaching the rest of the atrium. (However, the scars may take from two to three months to fully form.) Once the scars form, any A-Fib impulses are blocked, thereby electrically "disconnecting" them or "isolating" them from the heart. This allows the Sinus Node to once again control the heart rhythm, and a normal heart rhythm is restored.

The success of an ablation or isolation is tested by trying to artificially "induce" A-Fib again. If A-Fib can be induced, additional possible trigger areas are ablated.

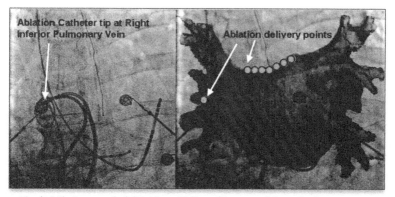

Visual 26: The image on the left is taken with X-rays (fluoroscopy). Several catheters are seen in the heart. When the CT image is added to the frame (shown at the right), the location of the pulmonary veins can be clearly identified.

During the procedure one can be completely unconscious (general anesthesia) or under conscious sedation (somewhat awake). Even under conscious sedation, a PVI is a relatively painless procedure because there are no nerve endings in the smooth tissue of the heart and veins. (However, some people do report experiencing pain during a PVI).

A catheter ablation usually takes up to three to four hours from beginning to end.

Over time, catheter ablation of A-Fib has gained acceptance as a first-line treatment option.[152] But, many doctors won't consider a catheter ablation for an A-Fib patient unless their symptoms are severe enough to interfere with their quality of life, and they have failed or been intolerant of at least one antiarrhythmic medication.

A Pulmonary Vein Isolation catheter ablation procedure can be repeated, if necessary.

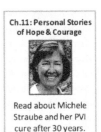

Ch.11: Personal Stories of Hope & Courage

Read about Michele Straube and her PVI cure after 30 years.

Other Locations of A-Fib Signals

While the pulmonary veins are the leading source of A-Fib signals, they aren't the only sources. Your doctor may discover signals originating from elsewhere in your heart such as from the Left Atrial Appendage, the Left Atrium Roof or the Septum to name a few.

For patients with Long-standing Persistent A-Fib (episodes lasting more than a year), 20% or more of the triggers are dispersed throughout different parts of the atrium, and are different for every patient.[153] The catheter ablation procedure for these patients will usually start with ablation of the pulmonary veins followed by the ablation of these additional signal locations.

Signals called Complex Fractionated Atrial Electrograms (CFAEs) are increasingly being used as targets of catheter ablation. They are low voltage electrical signals with very short cycle lengths used to identify areas in the heart that need to be ablated. CFAEs are often ablated in addition to, and after the ablation of the pulmonary veins.[154]

Isolation Techniques

If you are experiencing A-Fib symptoms during your procedure, it's relatively easy for the doctors to determine where the A-Fib signals are coming from and to ablate (remove) or isolate them. The challenge for doctors is with patients whose A-Fib is intermittent and who are not in A-Fib during the procedure. Doctors have strategies for this situation.

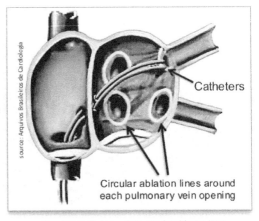

source: Arquivos Brasileiros de Cardiologia

Catheters

Circular ablation lines around each pulmonary vein opening

Visual 27: Catheters create circular ablation lines around each pulmonary vein opening.

One strategy replaces the need to identify specific signal origins. Instead, circular radiofrequency (RF) ablation lines are made around each pulmonary vein opening (called "Circumferential Ablation"). This isolates the pulmonary veins from the rest of the heart and prevents any pulses from these veins getting through.

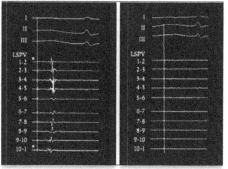

Visual 28: Pulmonary Vein Potentials, (L) Initial electrogram measurements show PV potentials, (R) Post-therapy all PV potentials eliminated.

Another strategy uses Pulmonary Vein Potentials. A "potential" is an electrical charge or energy—like the energy stored in your car battery. Even if your car isn't running, you can still measure 12 volts "potential" at the battery.

Similarly, in your heart any potential(s) in a pulmonary vein can be measured and pinpointed, even if you aren't in A-Fib. When the area is ablated or isolated with a radiofrequency (RF) catheter, the potential disappears or is disconnected. Like taking the battery out of your car, removing this potential eliminates your A-Fib.

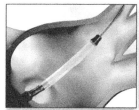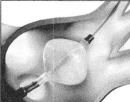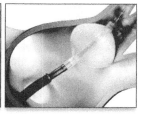

Visual 29: Arctic Front® Cardiac CryoAblation Catheter by Medtronic
(L) Closed; (C) Inflate and Position; (R) Occlude and Ablate.

An alternative to the use of an RF catheter is a Cryo (freezing) balloon catheter. Typical RF catheters make circular ablation lines around pulmonary vein openings, point-by-point, which requires significant operator skill and is time consuming. But the CryoBalloon catheter creates a circumferential lesion with a single "freezing" application.

The balloon inflates and is pressed up against the pulmonary vein opening. The balloon fills with coolant which makes the balloon stick to the PV opening until the tissue is ablated.

FDA-approved in late 2010, clinical trials showed the CryoBalloon was faster, easier to use, and appears to be safer than RF ablation.[155] Currently the CryoBalloon catheter is not approved for making linear lesions that may be required in patients with right or left atrial flutter or persistent A-Fib.[156] But cryo linear lesions can be made point-by-point with the FDA-approved Cryo Freezor MAX Arctic Front catheter.

Ch.11: Personal Stories of Hope & Courage

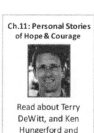

Read about Terry DeWitt, and Ken Hungerford and CryoBalloon ablations.

Post-Procedure Recovery

Your post-op hospital stay may be one to three days. Or, with an uncomplicated ablation, you might go home in four–six hours (this is because most complications occur in the first few hours following the procedure).[157]

It takes several weeks for the ablation scars to fully form. Therefore, your doctor allows a two-to-three month "recovery" or "blanking" period before deciding if your ablation was successful.

It is common to experience A-Fib episodes early during the recovery period (the first two to six weeks). Rarely, Atrial Fibrillation may be worse for a few weeks after the procedure and may be related to inflammation where the lesions were created. In most patients, these episodes subside within one to three months.

At your three month post-procedure check-up, you and your doctor will discuss whether you need to continue any medication. Subsequent follow-up evaluations may be every 6 to 12 months.

Outcome Results and Recurrence Rates

Success rates have been reported in the range of 70%–85% for patients with occasional (Paroxysmal) A-Fib. [158, 159, 160, 161] (Since catheter ablation for A-Fib is a relatively new procedure, research data beyond five years continues to be acquired and studied.)

> ❖ "Up to 80% of patients were A-Fib free, i.e., in normal sinus rhythm with or without the use of medication."

The most recent worldwide survey of over 16,000 patients undergoing catheter ablations covered a four-year period. Up to 80% of patients were A-Fib free, i.e., in normal sinus rhythm (NSR) with or without the use of medication (approximately 70% were in NSR _and_ free of medication).[162]

About a third of patients needed an additional catheter ablation. This increased the overall success rate to over 87% for patients with Paroxysmal or Persistent A-Fib. For those with Long-standing Persistent A-Fib, success rates were not as high.

Recurrence rates: There is increasing evidence that a successful PVI for A-Fib isn't always permanent.[163, 164] Recent studies indicate a 7%–9% chance of A-Fib returning each year out to five years.[165, 166, 167, 168]

Ch.11: Personal Stories of Hope & Courage

Read about Warren Welsh, A-Fib free after two PVIs.

If your heart heals itself and generates A-Fib signals again, this doesn't mean your PVI procedure failed. You may only have a few brief A-Fib episodes; or you may be happily free of A-Fib for years, and then just need a "touch-up" PVI procedure to put you back into normal sinus rhythm.

Additionally, those not "cured" by their PVI, may nonetheless be significantly improved with a better quality of life. They may have fewer or less intense attacks of A-Fib; medications that didn't work before may now control the A-Fib. But for some, there may not be any noticeable improvement at all.

Significant Side Benefit of Catheter Ablation

Even if your A-Fib recurs after catheter ablation, a new study reveals a significant side benefit. Catheter ablation patients have a significantly lower risk of death, stroke, and dementia compared to A-Fib patients who did not have an ablation. And better yet, after an ablation, these risk rates return to the levels of those with no A-Fib at all.[169]

Definition of Success

You may be asking yourself, just how is "success" defined?

Dr. Pierre Jais, from the French Bordeaux Group, defines success as "restoring a patient to normal sinus rhythm without dependence on any medications."[170] Another definition is freedom from A-Fib in the absence of antiarrhythmic drug therapy.[171]

> ❖ *You may be asking yourself, just how is "success" defined?*

In other words, the <u>best</u> outcome is to be A-Fib free <u>without</u> use of drugs. But for many A-Fib patients, an <u>acceptable</u> outcome is to be A-Fib free even <u>with</u> the use of antiarrhythmic drugs.

Energy Sources and Catheters

One key to a successful ablation is delivering the precise amount of energy necessary to ablate the tissue without damaging surrounding structures. This is as much art as it is science, which explains why so many A-Fib patients select a doctor and/or medical center with a record of high-volume catheter ablations. Through experience these doctors have higher success rates and fewer complications.

Another key to a successful ablation is creating scar tissue (transmural lesions) that reliably and completely penetrates heart tissue.

Various energy sources may be used; but the only two approved by the FDA are heat, in the form of high-frequency radio waves, called Radio Frequency (RF) Ablation, and cold energy known as Cryoablation.[172]

In the future, other energy sources may be used including microwave (electromagnetic radiation), focused ultrasound (acoustic energy) and laser.

Energy sources are often combined with new catheter tip ablation devices.

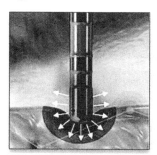 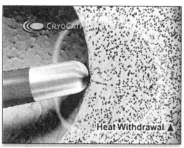

Visual 30: (L) Radio Frequency (RF) catheter; (R) Cryo tip removes heat (rather than adding cold).

There are now irrigated tips, circular catheters, mesh catheters and balloon catheters in addition to traditional catheter tips. With the balloon catheter, energy is delivered to a broad area with a single application.

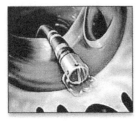 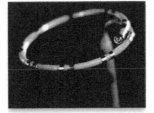 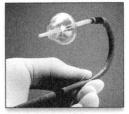

Visual 31: (L) ThermoCool irrigated tip catheter; (C) LASSO 2515 Variable Circular Mapping catheter from Biosense Webster; (R) CardioFocus balloon catheter steerable sheath.

When to Consider Pulmonary Vein Isolation

If you cannot tolerate rate control or antiarrhythmic medications, or they are ineffective, you should definitely consider catheter ablation (Pulmonary Vein Isolation). In addition, if you don't want to be on medications for the rest of your life, or your A-Fib symptoms are persistent and severely affect the quality of your life, talk to your EP about a PVI.

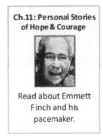

Ch.11: Personal Stories of Hope & Courage

Read about Emmett Finch and his pacemaker.

AV NODE ABLATION WITH PACEMAKER

Most A-Fib patients should exhaust all other treatments for Atrial Fibrillation before considering an AV Node Ablation. This procedure significantly diminishes or eliminates your A-Fib symptoms. It does not, however, eliminate or cure your A-Fib, and does not remove the risk of stroke. In addition, it leaves you pacemaker-dependent for the rest of your life.

The AV Node is the normal pathway that lets heartbeats from the top chambers of the heart make their way to the bottom chambers. Each normal heartbeat starts in the right atrium where a specialized group of cells (the Sinus Node) generates an electrical signal that travels down a single electrical road (the AV Node) that connects the atria to the ventricles below. By ablating or eliminating this AV Node, your Atrial Fibrillation signals can't get to the ventricles—which *does*

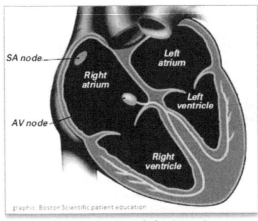

Visual 32: Sinus Node (SA) and AV Node.

stop your heart from racing. But for your heart to beat, you *must* have a permanent pacemaker implanted in your heart.

Post-Procedure Concerns

Patients with occasional (Paroxysmal) A-Fib who have an AV Node Ablation often develop Long-standing Persistent A-Fib afterwards.[173]

After this procedure, you still have A-Fib and have to forever take anticoagulants to prevent stroke. Because you still have A-Fib, over time your A-Fib may decrease mental abilities and lead to dementia.[174] In addition, when you eliminate the AV Node, there is a risk of sudden death because of the ventricles beating too fast.[175]

When to Consider an AV Node Ablation with Insertion of a Pacemaker

After exhausting all other options (i.e., Pulmonary Vein Isolations and/or Maze type surgery), consider an AV Node Ablation if you have persistent symptoms with an elevated heart rate (130 to 140 bpm) that goes even higher with exercise or exertion; or you are 80 years old or older. In either case you must be willing to live with a pacemaker and continue to take anticoagulants to prevent stroke.

From a patient's point of view this is a procedure of last resort, but it does work. Patients report an improved quality of life, being able to return to physical activities (i.e., playing 18 holes of golf) enjoyed before their A-Fib was symptomatic.

MAZE SURGERIES

The Classic Cox-Maze Operations

Unlike catheter ablation which enters the heart from inside your body, the Cox-Maze operations are "open-heart" surgeries where the breastbone is cracked open and large incisions made in the sternum. The heart is stopped and the patient placed on a heart-lung machine (cardiopulmonary bypass).

In the 1980s Classic Cox-Maze surgeries (Cox-Maze I and Cox-Maze II) the surgeon worked on the left and right atria making extensive linear incisions to create electrically isolated segments. The incisions generated scar tissues that

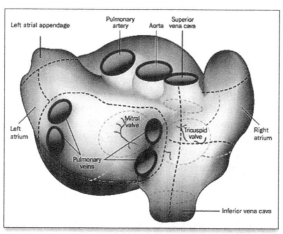

Visual 33: Surgical Maze pattern of lesions.

served as barriers, trapping abnormal electric signals. This "maze" of barricades confined the electrical impulses to defined pathways leading to the AV Node. The atria continued to be activated by a regular signal from the Sinus Node. In addition, the Left Atrial Appendage (the source of most blood clots) was removed.

The Cox-Maze surgery is a technically difficult, though highly successful technique for the treatment of A-Fib.

Cox-Maze III

Over time the Maze surgery has been revised and improved. Today's Cox-Maze III surgery, first performed in 1992, remains highly invasive (open chest), and requires cardiopulmonary bypass, and, when performed alone, can be associated with significant complications. Not all patients are healthy enough to endure this operation.

However, if the Cox-Maze III is performed along with another cardiac surgery, for example a mitral valve repair, it is not associated with any higher mortality or complication rate than that of the concurrent surgery.[176] As a simultaneous procedure, the Cox-Maze III has a greater than 90% A-Fib cure rate ten years after the surgery.[177]

The Cox-Maze III is sometimes called the "traditional Maze", the "cut and sew maze", or simply the "Maze." It is an extremely complex surgery; therefore, few surgeons do it.

The Cox-Maze is usually limited to those who require cardiac surgery for another serious heart condition.

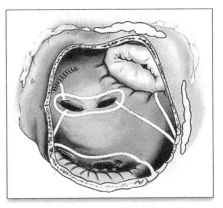

Visual 34: Maze surgery pattern of RF lesions.

Cox-Maze IV

The newest refinement of the Maze is the Cox-Maze IV. While it remains an open chest operation with cardiopulmonary bypass and a full Cox-Maze lesion set, the surgeon's scalpel and most of the "cut and sew" incisions are replaced with linear ablation lesions (scars) created either with radiofrequency energy (heat) or cryothermal energy (freezing).[178]

Energy is delivered through a clamp equipped with electrodes imbedded in the jaws. Results compare with the Cox-Maze III surgery.[179]

Success rates and recurrence are similar to a PVI ablation procedure.[180]

The Cox-Maze III and Cox-Maze IV operations aren't often used because of the risks associated with open-heart surgery, the danger of bleeding from the incisions, the pain, discomfort and prolonged convalescence from the operation, and the resulting reduced atrial function due to the incisions.

However, if you have to undergo open-heart surgery for another heart problem (such as coronary artery bypass and valve repair or replacement), you may want the Cox-Maze operation performed at the same time for your A-Fib.

The Minimally-Invasive Cox-Maze IV

A variation of the Cox-Maze IV replaces the "open chest" access (through the breast bone) with small incisions between the ribs. The patient is still placed on cardiopulmonary bypass; the full set of linear ablation lesions are created either with RF or cryothermal energy, and the Left Atrial Appendix is removed. This variation is called the "Minimally Invasive Cox IV."[181]

The Cox-Maze operations <u>cannot</u> be repeated if unsuccessful in eliminating the A-Fib signals.

> **Ch.11: Personal Stories of Hope & Courage**
>
> Read about Sheri Weber and her Minimally Invasive Cox IV Maze surgery.

Mini-Maze Surgery

In recent years, surgeons have developed a modification of the Cox-Maze called the Mini-Maze, short for "Minimal Maze."

Unlike the Cox-Maze III and Cox-Maze IV, the Mini-Maze surgery (such as the Wolf Mini-Maze) is a "keyhole" procedure performed on a beating heart without opening the chest, and without the need for cardiopulmonary bypass (heart-lung machine). It focuses on isolating the pulmonary veins.

Small incisions are made in the chest between the ribs. The heart's double-walled sac (the pericardium) is opened to access the heart. The incisions allow the surgeon to insert and maneuver the surgical instruments—an ablation device and an endoscope (a flexible tube with a small camera and light to view the heart).

Working in a specific pattern, a clamp with radiofrequency (or other energy source) is used to make a series of lesions to ablate (burn) the tissue and electrically isolate the pulmonary veins (where most

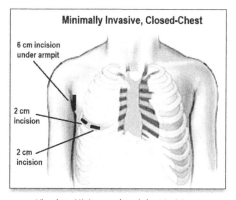

Visual 35: Mini-maze closed chest incisions.

A-Fib triggers originate). To be effective, the ablation lesions must be "transmural" (penetrate all the way from the outside of the heart to the inside).

A current drawback to the Wolf Mini-Maze surgery is that it can't always reach or block every area of the heart where A-Fib signals can originate such as the septum, or, in the case of most Atrial Flutter, the right atrium.

Most Mini-Maze operations take three to four hours, with post-operative hospital stay averaging three to four days. Unlike the other Maze operations, Mini-Maze surgeries are being used with "younger" patients (under 60 years of age) with Lone Atrial Fibrillation (no underlying heart disease).[182]

Variations of the Mini-Maze include the Totally Thoracoscopic (TT) Maze, the Five-Box Thoracoscopic Maze, and the Dallas Extended Lesion Set. In addition to isolating the pulmonary veins, each applies a select set of lesions to the left atrium. But these lesions do not duplicate the Cox-Maze lesion set.

Topics to Discuss With the Cardiac Surgeon

Newer Mini-Maze surgeries, such as the Totally Thoracoscopic (TT) Maze, the Five-Box Thoracoscopic Maze, and the Dallas Extended Lesion Set, create ablation lines on the left atrium. Circulation, nerve signal pathways, heart muscle fibers, transport function, etc. may be affected. Researchers don't know if this extensive scarring is necessary or appropriate for all cases of A-Fib.

Ch.11: Personal Stories of Hope & Courage

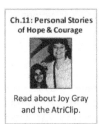

Read about Daniel Doane and his TT Mini-Maze.

In addition, the Mini-Maze operations customarily staple shut or close off the Left Atrial Appendage where A-Fib-related blood clots usually originate. This greatly reduces the risk of stroke if still in A-Fib after the surgery. But the surgical success rate for fully closing off the Left Atrial Appendage is disappointingly low. A study by surgeon Ralph Damiano, Jr., MD, found both suture and stapler methods had extraordinarily low success rates with clear evidence of the inadequacy of these techniques. [183]

However, the recently developed Atritech AtriClip device makes it easier for surgeons to close off the Left Atrial Appendage. To implant the clip, the surgeon positions the rectangular-shaped device around the LAA and then closes it like a clamp. The blood no longer flows into or out of the LAA.

Ch.11: Personal Stories of Hope & Courage

Read about Joy Gray and the AtriClip.

While removal of the Left Atrial Appendage is the current practice in Mini-Maze (and Cox-Maze) surgeries, some question the need or benefit. The LAA functions like a reservoir or decompression chamber to prevent surges of blood in the left atrium when the mitral valve is closed. Without it, there is increased pressure on the pulmonary veins and left atrium. Also, closing off the LAA will somewhat decrease the amount of blood pumped by the heart. And the Left Atrial Appendage is a major endocrine organ (i.e. hormone secreting gland); removal may increase the tendency to become dehydrated. These issues may be of special concern for younger people and those with physical lifestyles.

So should you or shouldn't you close off the LAA? For those at risk for clot formation, the reduced risk of stroke may outweigh the above concerns. Conversely, those with low risk of clot formation, including those with lone A-Fib or Atrial Flutter, may not want to remove the LAA. [184]

Questions When Considering a Mini-Maze

When considering a Mini-Maze, you should ask your cardiac surgeon:

- Would a catheter ablation fix my A-Fib without the added risks of heart surgery (such as Pulmonary Vein Isolation)?
- If I choose a Mini-Maze surgery, how extensive are the ablation lines on the Left Atrium? Will this scarring permanently affect other heart functions (I.e., circulation, nerve signal pathways, heart muscle fibers, transport function, etc.)?
- Is this amount of ablation lines necessary to fix my type of A-Fib?

- Are these ablation lines limited to the pulmonary veins? What if A-Fib signals are coming from other areas of my heart?
- Will you staple shut or close off the Left Atrial Appendage? Is this necessary if you expect me to be A-Fib free after the surgery?
- If the LAA will be closed off, what technique will you use (i.e., suture or stapler methods, or Atritech AtriClip)? How do you know if you have successfully closed off the entire LAA?

These are important issues to discuss with your medical advisors before choosing a Mini-Maze surgery to cure your A-Fib.

Outcome Results and Recurrence Rates

The Mini-Maze surgery is a relatively new procedure. There is little research data beyond five years.

The most recent research studies followed patients 6–12 months post-op. Of patients with Paroxysmal A-Fib, up to 87% were in normal sinus rhythm with or without use of medication (65–72% were in NSR *and* free of medication); and 47–54% of Persistent and Long-standing Persistent A-Fib patients were in NSR (with or without use of medication).[185, 186, 187]

As with catheter-based interventions, patients with recent onset Paroxysmal (newly diagnosed, occasional) atrial fibrillation enjoy greater success rates than patients with Persistent or Long-standing Persistent.[188]

Recurrence rates: A-Fib symptoms returned in about 35%–40% of cases within 6–12 months following surgery.[189, 190]

Note: "Recurrence" doesn't necessarily mean your Mini-Maze was a failure. A few transient A-Fib episodes after your recovery period may have little impact on your quality of life; or your A-Fib might return after several delightfully A-Fib free years.

Comparison of Mini-Maze and PVI

In principle, the Wolf Mini-Maze surgery is similar to a Pulmonary Vein Isolation ablation (PVI). The goal of both is to isolate the Pulmonary Vein openings. But whereas the cardiac surgeon makes several chest incisions and ablates from outside the heart, the electrophysiologist (EP) makes a small incision in the groin for the catheter and ablates from inside the heart.

There are a few important differences. If more areas of your heart need to be ablated or isolated, catheter ablations can be tailored to the different locations of A-Fib signals, including ablating for Atrial Flutter if needed. The Wolf Mini-Maze surgical lesion sets are presently "one size fits all." They only isolate the Pulmonary Veins and don't normally access other parts of the heart to ablate other sources of A-Fib signals. The Mini-Maze does not address Atrial Flutter which usually comes from the Right Atrium.

Also, the Mini-Maze customarily staples shut or closes off the Left Atrial Appendage. The PVI procedure does not.

Note: if you have Atrial Flutter in addition to Atrial Fibrillation, today's PVI procedures routinely include ablation of the right atrium (the location of most cases of Atrial Flutter) thereby fixing two problems with one procedure. But if you have a Mini-Maze surgery, you will need a subsequent ablation procedure to treat your Atrial Flutter.

When to Consider Cox-Maze Surgery or Mini-Maze Surgery

Consider a traditional Maze (Cox-Maze III or IV) if you have to undergo open-heart surgery for another heart problem; the Cox-Maze operation can be performed at the same time with no additional health risk, and with high success rates.

Consider a Mini-Maze surgery if you:

- are allergic to blood thinners (i.e., Coumadin) and therefore cannot undergo a catheter ablation (blood thinners are required for catheter ablation procedures but not for Mini-Maze Surgery)
- have a history of stroke
- are very overweight (morbidly obese) and don't qualify for a catheter ablation (due to difficulty getting clear fluoroscopic images and subsequent risk of greater doses of radiation).

If you have a simple case of new (recent onset) A-Fib, the Mini Maze operation may work for you. It is not as successful for more complicated cases of A-Fib.

The Mini-Maze operations <u>cannot</u> be repeated if unsuccessful in eliminating A-Fib signals.

PACEMAKERS AND IMPLANTABLE CARDIOVERTER DEFIBRILLATORS (ICD)

Pacemakers and Implantable Cardioverter Defibrillators (ICDs) are devices used to address heart conditions by delivering electrical impulses to the heart when there is a rhythm problem. But a pacemaker and an ICD are designed for different purposes.

The pacemaker helps to regulate the heartbeat, keeping the rhythm stable; while an ICD is designed to "shock" the heart when it's beating dangerously fast or has stopped beating.

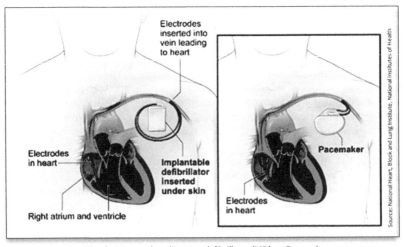

Visual 36: Internal cardioverter defibrillator (ICD) vs. Pacemaker.

Pacemakers

For those with A-Fib, a pacemaker is usually implanted only if your heart rate is too slow (for example, as a result of taking A-Fib medications) or if you have Sinus Node and/or Atrioventricular (AV) Node problems.[191]

In general, pacemakers are not very effective for controlling A-Fib.

Internal Cardioverter Defibrillators (ICD)

An Implantable Cardioverter Defibrillator (ICD) is similar to a pacemaker, but there are some important differences. When the heart beats too rapidly, or fibrillates instead of contracting strongly, or stops beating, an ICD sends electronic signals to the heart. These signals shock the heart into beating more slowly and pumping more effectively. The ICD acts as an internal version of the shock paddles used by physicians during an electrical cardioversion.

A defibrillator shock is painful, like being "kicked in the chest." Most people would rather have A-Fib than be shocked throughout the day and night. Also, it does not address the underlying problem or condition of your heart that causes your A-Fib.

This device is typically *not* used to treat Atrial Fibrillation.

SUMMARY

The good news for people with Atrial Fibrillation is that there are a greater range of treatment options and more effective treatments than ever before.

Cardioversion offers immediate, but short lived results. Pulmonary Vein Isolation procedures (PVIs) are comparatively low risk and achieve success rates of 70%-85% in curing occasional (Paroxysmal) A-Fib. A second catheter ablation, when appropriate, can increase the success rate.

The Cox-Maze surgeries offer high success rates when performed along with surgery for another heart problem.

The Mini-Maze Surgery is similar in principle to a PVI catheter ablation. The cardiac surgeon isolates the pulmonary veins from outside the heart, while the electrophysiologist isolates from inside the heart. If one is allergic to blood thinners, the Mini-Maze Surgery should be considered.

For A-Fib patients who have tried all other options, an AV Node Ablation with Pacemaker may offer relief from A-Fib symptoms (but is not a cure, and the risk of stroke remains).

❖

Many of your fellow patients want answers to some of the same questions that may be on your mind at this point. In the next chapter we'll review frequently asked patient questions about the control and treatment of your A-Fib.

❖

CHAPTER EIGHT

FAQs About A-Fib Treatments

We've covered a lot of information about the various A-Fib treatments. Based on over ten years of working with A-Fib patients through our website (A-Fib.com), we have fielded thousands of questions—the same questions that may be on your mind at this point.

Here are the most frequently asked questions and answers regarding the control and treatment of A-Fib.

1. **Is Atrial Fibrillation curable? Or can you only treat or control it?**

    A-Fib is definitely curable. No matter how long you've had A-Fib, your goal should be a complete and permanent cure (restored to normal sinus rhythm without dependence on any medications). If your doctor is satisfied with only keeping your A-Fib "under control," we urge you to look for another doctor.

    Note: While you may not be eligible for all types of treatments and not all A-Fib procedures or surgeries are successful, your target goal, none the less, should still be a complete and permanent cure, i.e. a life free of A-Fib.

2. **Is there a diet I could follow which would cure my A-Fib?**

    Research hasn't identified a diet which would cure your A-Fib. In general, a healthy diet promotes your overall health and thereby possibly improves your A-Fib.

    Specifically, a heart-healthy diet includes proper levels of minerals called electrolytes. A-Fib patients are usually deficient in magnesium and potassium and may be consuming too much calcium. Have your doctor test for proper levels of magnesium, calcium and potassium. You may need to adjust your diet or use supplements to restore proper levels.

    In addition, consider identifying if you have any A-Fib "triggers." You may want to lessen or eliminate foods that appear to trigger your A-Fib, such as heavy alcohol consumption and stimulants (tea, chocolate, tobacco, MSG, sodas) to determine if that helps your condition.

    Keep a log or diary of what you consume along with the occurrences of your A-Fib episodes. Look for patterns; test for triggers. For example, if you suspect chocolate is a trigger, test its effect by not eating any for one or two weeks. Did you have fewer or less intense episodes? Test each potential trigger and adjust your diet as necessary.

3. **Are there exercises that will help eliminate my Atrial Fibrillation?**

    No. Research hasn't identified any exercises that would help eliminate your A-Fib. (Some people say they can come out of an A-Fib attack by bearing down hard using their diaphragm. Others report that exercise can often get them out of an A-Fib attack.)

4. *Should I monitor my heart rate?*

    If you want to monitor your heart rate, you can try an athlete's heart rate monitor available from sporting goods stores. They strap around your chest and transmit your heart rate to a special wrist watch. You can set it to sound an alarm if your pulse exceeds a certain rate.

5. *I like my Cardiologist, but he hasn't referred me to an Electrophysiologist. Should I ask for a second opinion?*

    Most definitely get a second opinion. An Electrophysiologist is a Cardiologist who specializes in heart rhythm problems. In fact, it's easy to find a local Electrophysiologist yourself. The web site of the Heart Rhythm Society has a feature called, *Finding a Heart Rhythm Specialist*. When you type in your State and City (or country), the site gives you a list of Electrophysiologists in your area. However, not all Electrophysiologists specialize in Atrial Fibrillation, so check under "Practice Information" and look for AF Ablation. *(See Chapter 10: Finding the Doctor for You).*

6. *I have a lot of extra beats and palpitations which are very disturbing and frightful. They seem to precede an A-Fib attack. What can or should I do about them?*

    Extra beats, called Premature Atrial Contractions (PACs) or Premature Ventricle Contractions (PVCs), are generally considered benign. Everybody gets them. But for people with A-Fib, PACs typically trigger A-Fib episodes.[192] Premature Ventricle Contractions (PVCs) may cause PACs, thereby also triggering A-Fib attacks.

    You may want to talk with your doctor about the "Pill-in-the-Pocket" treatment—use of an antiarrhythmic prescription drug taken when you get PACs. They may stop or shorten your A-Fib attacks.

7. *I have Paroxysmal (occasional) A-Fib. I'm worried my A-Fib may become chronic, which I know is harder to cure. How long do I have before it becomes permanent?*

    Odds are you have about one year.

    In a study of over 5,000 A-Fib patients, 54% of those on rate control meds went into Long-standing Persistent A-Fib within one year.[193] Therefore, you should aggressively seek to stop your A-Fib through either antiarrhythmic meds, or catheter ablation, or surgery.

    On the other hand, there are patients who've had Paroxysmal A-Fib for years and never progress to Persistent or Long-standing Persistent A-Fib.

8. *I'm getting by with my Atrial Fibrillation. With continuing improvements in Pulmonary Vein Isolation techniques, should I wait until a better technique is developed?*

    A-Fib is a progressive condition. In general, the longer you have it—the worse it gets. In a process called "remodeling," your heart may change physically and electrically if you have A-Fib long enough. It's important to be cured as reasonably soon as possible.

    With Pulmonary Vein Isolation procedures, you have a 70%–85% chance of being cured permanently (in cases of Paroxysmal A-Fib).[194] [195] The A-Fib symptoms of the other A-Fib patients are often significantly improved. (Those are pretty good odds.)

9. *I definitely have A-Flutter and possibly A-Fib as well. They want to do a Flutter-only ablation on me. Will that help me with both the Flutter and the A-Fib?*

Probably not. If you suffer from both A-Flutter and A-Fib and have a Flutter-only Ablation (ablation of the right atrium), the estimated success rate for also curing the A-Fib is only 5%–10 %.[196] You're usually wasting your time and undergoing needless risk to do a Flutter-only ablation when you also have A-Fib.

But what if you have Atrial Flutter and <u>not</u> A-Fib? "As many as half of all patients ablated for Flutter later develop A-Fib."[197] A research study suggests that anyone with only A-Flutter would be better served by an ablation of both the left and right atria instead of just the right atrium.[198] (While uncommon, some Atrial Flutter does originate from the left atrium.)

10. *What are the risks of a Pulmonary Vein Isolation (PVI) procedure? How do doctors protect patients from these risks?*

As a point of reference, the complication rate for the common Appendectomy is about 18%.[199] Catheter ablation has a complication rate of 1%–3%,[200] comparable to other routine, low-risk procedures such as Tubal Ligation (1%–2%).

A small percentage of PVI patients develop minor complications[201] such as bleeding and bruising at the groin (where the catheters are inserted). This is usually a temporary complication that resolves in two–three weeks.

About 2% of patients develop more serious or major complications[202] such as:

- *Stenosis. (Constriction or narrowing of the Pulmonary Vein openings reducing blood flow from the lungs to the heart.) Stenosis is increasingly rare because most ablations are now performed outside the Pulmonary Vein openings. In addition, stents can often open up the swelled areas. (Ask your doctor or medical center about their rate of Stenosis.)*

- *Stroke. During an ablation, you are administered a more powerful anticoagulant like heparin to prevent formation of a clot. If a clot does form, a medication like TPA (Tissue Plasminogen Activator) is used to dissolve it. The risk of a stroke during an ablation in some centers is less than one in 200 (less than 0.5%).[203] That's compared to a 2%–8% chance of stroke from cardiac surgery.[204]*

- *Tamponade. (Blood leaking into the sac around the heart from a catheter puncture.) A catheter puncture of the heart is rare and relates to the skill and experience of the ablation doctor. If this happens, blood must be drawn out of the Pericardium Sac, sometimes by surgery. While it can be fatal, once treated and the puncture heals, there is usually no lasting damage.*

- *Atrial-Esophageal Fistula. A very rare complication (less than one in over 1000 cases) that is often fatal. A Fistula is an abnormal duct or passage formed after RF heat damages the esophagus during a PVI, resulting in the heart leaking blood into the esophagus.*

  Doctors are aware of this danger to the esophagus and use many techniques to prevent Atrial-Esophageal Fistula including:

  - ➢ Low RF power when ablating in the back of the heart
  - ➢ Temperature monitoring using a probe from within the esophagus
  - ➢ Use of barium paste in the esophagus to aid in imaging and avoiding it
  - ➢ Use of Cryo ablation which eliminates possible heat damage to the esophagus
  - ➢ Use of Proton Pump Inhibitors for two–three weeks after an ablation to prevent ulceration (This is perhaps the easiest way to prevent Atrial-Esophageal Fistula, and one that patients can use themselves without a prescription. But check with your doctor first.)

As with any medical procedure, there is always the unforeseen, such as allergic reactions to medications or anesthesia, risk of infection, valve damage, or heart attack.

Be assured that doctors and staff monitor you very closely and are prepared to deal with emergencies and complications.

Bottom-line: for most A-Fib patients, it's probably safer getting a PVI than not getting one. The long-term risks of living a lifetime in A-Fib and/or on antiarrhythmic drugs is potentially more damaging than the generally short-term risks of a Pulmonary Vein Isolation.

11. **What are the risks of a Cox-Maze or Mini-Maze surgery?**

Both the Cox-Maze III and Cox-Maze IV operations are major heart surgeries. In general, minor complications associated with any heart surgery are temporary and easily treated and include nausea and vomiting, minor infections, minor bleeding or bruising, abnormal or painful scar formation, allergic skin reaction to tape, dressings, or latex, skin numbness and lingering pain at the incision cites.[205]

More serious but less frequent complications include risks such as stroke or heart attack, nerve damage, serious bleeding, lung problems including fluid buildup, kidney failure, allergic reaction to medication, anesthesia-related problems, and loss of life.[206]

COX-MAZE III

The Cox-Maze III is major open-chest surgery involving general anesthesia, heart lung bypass, cutting into the heart and sewing it back up, and cutting out the Left Atrial Appendage. Specific complications may include the need for a permanent pacemaker in about three of 100 cases (3.2%)[207], swelling and inflammation in the mid-chest area called mediastinitis (a life-threatening condition affecting 1%–2% of patients[208]), and sometimes a second operation to correct for complications. The mortality rate is about three out of 200 cases (1.4%).[209]

COX-MAZE IV

The Cox-Maze IV is a newer version of the Cox-Maze III with less cutting into the heart. Access to the heart can be through the ribs instead of through the breastbone. The Cox-Maze IV has approximately the same risks and possible complications as other major heart surgeries.

MINI-MAZE SURGERIES

In addition to the risks associated with normal heart surgery, the various Mini-Maze surgeries, though less invasive, still have their own set of risks and possible complications.

- *Deflating and re-inflating the lungs:* In most Mini-Maze surgeries the lungs are alternatively deflated and re-inflated to position the ablation clamp around each pulmonary vein. For older patients and others whose lungs are less elastic, the lungs may not properly re-inflate. Ventilators may have to be used during surgery to pump the lungs. This can damage lung tissue. If the lungs do re-inflate properly, one can still have weeks-long coughing spells, coughing up blood, etc.

  If a lung doesn't function properly, a temporary lung bypass machine may be used. The Extracorporeal Membrane Oxygenation (ECMO) unit carries blood out of the body so that a filter can remove carbon dioxide and re-infuse oxygen into the blood, and can be used until lung function is sufficiently recovered. This involves some risk, requires blood thinners to avoid clots, and can potentially lead to additional infection. An added risk is that ECMO machines are not available in all hospitals.

- *Difficulty making transmural lesions:* Making reliable lesions that completely penetrate the heart tissue isn't always easy to do from outside the heart (due to the cooling effects of circulating blood and variations in thickness and ridges within the heart tissue).

- *No mapping for verification:* Currently most Mini-Maze surgeries don't map inside the heart to verify if a particular lesion set is effective, i.e., transmural. (The exception is the new "Hybrid" procedures where surgeons and EPs simultaneously work on the same patient.)

- *Post-operation pain: Like any surgery, post-op pain is a concern.* Note: The pain associated with the access incisions between the ribs usually goes away in a few weeks.

Be assured that doctors and staff monitor you very closely, and are prepared to deal with emergencies and complications.

12. **How long does it take before I know the procedure or surgery was a success?**

Some people will be in perfect sinus rhythm after a catheter ablation (PVI) procedure or surgery.

But, your doctor will allow a two to three month "recovery" or "blanking" period before deciding if the ablation or surgery was successful. For most of us, it usually takes several months for the ablation scars or lesions to heal and for our heart to learn to beat normally again.

Don't be discouraged if you experience A-Fib episodes early during your recovery period. It's quite common. These episodes usually subside within one to three months. Doctors sometimes help this process by prescribing antiarrhythmic meds for a month or longer, or you may have to be electrocardioverted to be restored to normal sinus rhythm. You may also have to continue to take warfarin (Coumadin) for a while.

13. Will my A-Fib eventually return over time, or am I permanently cured?

Compared to other treatments for A-Fib such as drug therapy or cardioversion, ablation and surgery are currently a patient's only hope of a permanent cure. But there is increasing evidence that a successful ablation or surgery for A-Fib isn't always permanent. There is a tendency for ablated heart tissue to heal itself and start producing A-Fib signals again. But if this happens, it usually occurs within the first six months following your ablation or surgery.

Recurrence rates: After a successful PVI ablation, studies indicate a 7%–9% chance of A-Fib returning each year out to five years. (There is little data beyond five years since PVI catheter ablation is a relatively new procedure.)[210, 211, 212, 213] Cox-Maze IV recurrence rates are similar to a PVI ablation procedure.[214] For the Mini-Maze, recent studies showed A-Fib symptoms returned in about 35%–40% of cases within 6–12 months following surgery.[215, 216]

14. I have a defective Mitral Valve. Is it causing my A-Fib? Should I have my Mitral Valve fixed first before the A-Fib?

Mitral Valve problems seem to be related to A-Fib, possibly because the extra strain a defective Mitral Valve puts on the heart may cause stretching and put extra pressure on the Pulmonary Vein openings where most A-Fib originates. However, fixing your defective Mitral Valve isn't a guarantee of curing A-Fib. Once the A-Fib signals in your heart have been activated, they may continue firing after your Mitral Valve is fixed.

If your doctors are planning open-heart surgery to fix your Mitral Valve, you may want a Cox-Maze operation at the same time to fix your A-Fib. But bear in mind, the Cox-Maze operations are stressful for your heart and your body.

If considering a PVI, check into having it done first, that is, *before* your open-heart surgery. Some EPs will not do a PVI if you have an artificial Mitral Valve, because of the risk of blood clots and the risk of damaging the artificial Mitral Valve.

SUMMARY

From questions about diet and exercise, to answers about Pulmonary Vein Isolation and surgery. Did we answer some of the questions on your mind at this point and maybe some you didn't know you wanted to ask?

With those questions answered, are you ready to map out the path to your cure? In Part III we help you find the right doctor and point you in the right direction to achieve a life free of the burden of A-Fib.

❖

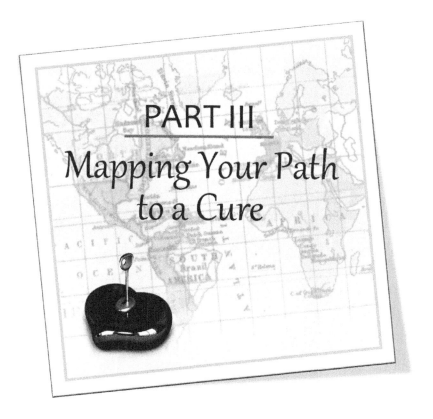

PART III

Mapping Your Path
to a Cure

❖

"I no longer live in the A-Fib shadow and no longer take the drugs.
My life is back. I no longer have to be content with less.
All is now quiet. ... Life is good."
Robert Dell
Free of A-Fib since 2002

❖

CHAPTER NINE

"Which Is the Best A-Fib Treatment Plan For Me?"

In this chapter we offer you treatment plan guidelines. We list the types of A-Fib the way patients themselves describe their A-Fib.

Keep in mind that Paroxysmal, Persistent, and Long-standing Persistent forms of Atrial Fibrillation often require very individualized treatment approaches.[217] A "one size fits all" strategy may not be the best option for your particular type of A-Fib. Your best A-Fib treatment option(s) is ultimately a decision only you and your doctor can make.

Note: Back in Chapter 7, we defined a successful cure as restoring a patient to normal sinus rhythm without dependence on any medications,[218] or freedom from A-Fib in the absence of antiarrhythmic drug therapy.[219]

Your best outcome, therefore, is to be A-Fib free without use of drugs. But for many A-Fib patients, an acceptable outcome is to be A-Fib free even with the use of antiarrhythmic drugs.

In this chapter, it's not necessary to read all the recommendations. Choose the statement(s) most closely related to your A-Fib, then read about your possible treatment options.

1. **My A-Fib just started.**

   New cases (recent onset) A-Fib may be helped by Electrical Cardioversion and/or Chemical Cardioversion. Doctors may be able to shock your heart back to beating normally; then, along with several months of antiarrhythmic meds, train your heart to stay in normal sinus rhythm. Ideally after this treatment, your heart won't go back into A-Fib. But don't delay. This treatment seems to work best in Recent Onset A-Fib.

   Note: Don't rely on Cardioversion for ongoing treatment of your A-Fib. While Cardioversion restores regular heart rhythm in more than 95 percent of patients, "50 to 75 percent of patients eventually develop Atrial Fibrillation again."[220]

2. **I have occasional (paroxysmal) A-Fib but with no symptoms (Silent A-Fib).**

   With "silent" A-Fib, you may be feeling okay. Your doctors may have discovered your A-Fib during a routine examination before you were aware of anything wrong.

   If you've had A-Fib for a while, an Electrical Cardioversion may not be successful in getting you back into normal sinus rhythm. But it may be worth a try.

   Another option is to just live with the A-Fib if symptoms don't affect you very much.

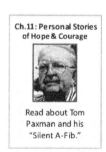

Ch.11: Personal Stories of Hope & Courage

Read about Tom Paxman and his "Silent A-Fib."

Talk with your doctor about whether or not you should be on blood thinners—with "silent" A-Fib you are still at risk of an A-Fib stroke. Your doctor may also prescribe Rate Control medications to make sure your heart doesn't beat too fast.

However, just living with A-Fib may eventually cause you problems. Over time A-Fib tends to "remodel" your heart, i.e., to stretch and weaken it, often leading to other heart problems and heart failure.[221] If your A-Fib worsens over the years, an enlarged atrium (over 55 mm in diameter) may limit your future treatment options. Also, over a prolonged period of time, A-Fib may lead to decreased mental abilities and even dementia, because blood isn't being pumped properly to the brain and other organs.

So if you choose to just live with your "silent" A-Fib, it's important to be closely monitored. Your atria should be measured regularly to see if they are being stretched and enlarged. Your cognitive abilities should be tracked over time, as well.

Because your A-Fib is "silent" with infrequent episodes, the use of antiarrhythmic medications, a Pulmonary Vein Isolation procedure or surgery may not be justified. (Many doctors won't perform a PVI on someone with relatively few A-Fib symptoms.)

On the positive side, you may be able to live for years with occasional "silent" A-Fib episodes which don't progress to anything worse.

3. *I have infrequent, short episodes of A-Fib.*

An Electrical Cardioversion (along with several months of antiarrhythmic meds to train your heart to stay in normal sinus rhythm) is an option worth trying. In general, Cardioversion has the best chance of success with new (early onset) A-Fib. (Most Cardioversion patients eventually develop Atrial Fibrillation again.)[222]

If your symptoms are bearable, another option is learning to live with your A-Fib. But this entails more than just putting up with A-Fib symptoms. You must also handle the psychological strain and fear of knowing an A-Fib attack is always possible. You have to decide if this is a treatment option that is acceptable to you.

Since your A-Fib episodes are relatively infrequent, a third option is taking antiarrhythmic meds which may keep your heart in normal sinus rhythm. Some patients with infrequent, short episodes have had success with the antiarrhythmic drug flecainide (brand name Tambocor) or the newer meds dofetilide (Tikosyn), Rythmol SR and dronedarone (Multaq). But be aware of possible unwanted side effects. Allow time for your body to adjust to the medications before you decide whether the side effects are acceptable or not.

And finally, a Pulmonary Vein Isolation (PVI) procedure has a good chance of curing you. However, many doctors and medical centers are hesitant to perform a PVI on someone with relatively infrequent A-Fib episodes. Be courageous. You may need to be very assertive and insist that you want a PVI and not a life on antiarrhythmic meds.

4. *I have paroxysmal (occasional) A-Fib but am in good health overall.*

    An Electrical Cardioversion may be effective for you, though it generally has the best chance of success with new (early onset) A-Fib. However, most Cardioversion patients eventually develop Atrial Fibrillation again.

    Antiarrhythmic meds may help in the short term, but they tend to lose their effectiveness over time. In general, don't expect an antiarrhythmic drug to be a permanent cure for your A-Fib.

    If seeking to cure your A-Fib rather than just "managing it", you should consider a Pulmonary Vein Isolation (PVI) procedure. Besides the Pulmonary Veins openings, a PVI can also ablate A-Fib signals coming from other areas of your heart. It's also the option that's the least invasive and traumatic to your body. The other option is one of the Mini-Maze surgeries which also ablates the pulmonary veins but accesses the outside of your heart through multiple chest incisions.

5. *I have paroxysmal (occasional) A-Fib but also have serious cardiac and other health problems.*

    For the A-Fib patient with structural heart disease, a drug therapy option is an antiarrhythmic drug such as Sotalol, Dofetilide, or Azimilide. They appear to be safer to use than other antiarrhythmic drugs.[223] (Amiodarone, probably the most effective antiarrhythmic med, often has serious side effects. The new drug dronedarone [Multaq] is similar to amiodarone but with less side effects.) But antiarrhythmics tend to lose their effectiveness over time and aren't usually a permanent cure for your A-Fib.

    Another option for you is a Pulmonary Vein Isolation (PVI) procedure which may also improve your overall heart health.

    But your chief priority must be to take care of your most serious heart and/or health problems first. If this requires cardiac surgery, you may want a surgeon to combine a Cox-Maze surgery with the other operation to correct your A-Fib at the same time. A Cox-Maze III or IV procedure is highly successful when performed along with another cardiac surgery.

6. *I have Persistent A-Fib; I have Long-standing Persistent A-Fib.*

    Patients with Persistent or Long-standing Persistent A-Fib often have multiple areas in the heart producing A-Fib signals. These A-Fib signal sources often have gotten stronger over time and are less likely to be affected by Electrical Cardioversion. Antiarrhythmic meds may also be less effective.

    The Pulmonary Vein Isolation (PVI) procedure's success rate with Persistent or Long-standing Persistent has greatly improved over the last few years. A recent study by the French Bordeaux group reported a 95% success rate in curing Long-standing Persistent A-Fib after two ablation procedures.[224] If you have Long-standing Persistent A-Fib, be prepared to have at least two ablation procedures. You also need to go to EPs more experienced in fixing Persistent A-Fib. But don't wait too long. Some centers do not accept patients who have had Long-standing Persistent A-Fib for over a year.

    Another option is the Cox-Maze IV. The recent developments in the Maze operations offer new hope[225] for those with Long-standing Persistent A-Fib.

(The Mini-Maze surgeries, in general, don't target specific A-Fib signal sources; so they aren't usually a good choice.)

7. **I have A-Fib. I'm allergic to blood thinners and have had a stroke.**

The need to avoid blood thinners rules out a Pulmonary Vein Isolation procedure. As a first option, consider Mini-Maze Surgery. A Mini-Maze is also a good option for those who have had a stroke, or who are more at risk of having a stroke during a catheter ablation.

Though not open-heart surgery, the Mini Maze operations are nevertheless very traumatic for the body.

One considered advantage of the Mini-Maze operations is that the Left Atrial Appendage (LAA), where blood clots usually originate, is cut out and/or stapled shut.[226] This greatly reduces the risk of stroke if still in A-Fib after the surgery.

The big drawback to the Wolf Mini-Maze surgery is it currently can't reach or block all areas of the heart, besides the pulmonary veins, where A-Fib signals may originate.

If you have a simple case of new (recent onset) A-Fib, the Mini-Maze operation may work for you. But it's not as successful for more complicated cases of A-Fib (when signals are generated by various other parts of the heart).

Your second option may be the Cox-Maze IV surgery. But an allergy to blood thinners may influence whether or not a surgeon takes your case, and may affect elements of the operation. While the Cox-Maze IV involves open-heart surgery and is more traumatic, it nonetheless has a high success rate in curing A-Fib.

8. **I know I'm seriously overweight. Doctors list me as "morbidly obese." But my heart starts racing whenever I try to exercise because of my A-Fib. What can I do? Should I get a Pulmonary Vein Isolation procedure (PVI), a Cox-Maze surgery or Mini-Maze?**

Electrophysiologists (EPs) may be reluctant to do a PVI in your case. Today's imaging systems have difficulty seeing through significant fat mass to get a clear picture of the heart.

As with A-Fib patients who have other major health problems, you may need specialized advice to safely lose weight before resolving your A-Fib (with special care not to further strain your heart). Consult with your EP to develop a target weight for you to qualify for a PVI.

Another option is for your EP to refer you to a Cardiothoracic Surgeon for Mini-Maze surgery. However, it is considered more traumatic, invasive, and risky than a PVI, and isn't a guaranteed success. (Make sure you discuss with the surgeon the risks of general anesthesia for someone who is overweight.)

9. **I'm 79 years old. Am I too old to be cured of my A-Fib?**

We've heard of people in their 90s who've had a successful A-Fib ablation. Your age and overall general health affect what treatments will work for you. The reason? Older patients tend to be more frail and prone to complications.

You will probably be offered antiarrhythmic meds as your only therapy choice. Surgical options may not be recommended for you.

Make sure you discuss a Pulmonary Vein Isolation procedure (PVI) with your electrophysiologist. (You may need to be courageous and persistent.)

Typically, your EP will want you to try antiarrhythmic meds for six months to a year before you can have a PVI. However, you can opt for a PVI right away, but you may have to be very assertive and insist that you don't want to take antiarrhythmic meds. (If you're over 80 years old, many centers will not accept you for a PVI. But not all centers have this policy.)

10. **I've had two failed left atrium ablations and have tried many different medications, but my A-Fib continues.**

You have several options to consider. First, a third ablation is a reasonable option for you, but you need to go to the best, most experienced A-Fib doctors you can find. You are a special case and deserve special treatment.

The high success rate of the Cox-Maze IV operation makes it another option for you.

A last option to consider is the "Ablation of the AV Node with Implanted Pacemaker" procedure. After this procedure you are still in A-Fib. You must still take blood thinners and probably rate control meds. But your ventricles are no longer affected by A-Fib. Even with a pacemaker, people report a better quality of life than when A-Fib made their heart race.

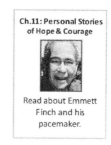

Ch.11: Personal Stories of Hope & Courage

Read about Emmett Finch and his pacemaker.

SUMMARY

In this chapter we reviewed the various patient scenarios for those with A-Fib. Did you find a description of your type of A-Fib? You should now have some specific treatment ideas and issues to discuss with your doctor.

❖

But which doctor is right for you? What type of doctor? In the next chapter we guide you through the steps to finding the right doctor for you.

❖

CHAPTER TEN
Finding the Doctor for You

In this chapter you'll learn about:
- The roles of cardiologists, electrophysiologists, and cardiothoracic surgeons
- How to find a specialist in heart rhythm disorders and abnormal heart rhythms
- Obtaining copies of your medical records
- Questions to help you find the right doctor for you

During your life with Atrial Fibrillation, you will probably consult with or be treated by several medical professionals including your family physician, various emergency room doctors, cardiologists, and other healthcare specialists. These doctors and their services include:

- *General Practitioner* (your family doctor): has overall responsibility for patient care and prescription of medication; may offer basic tests and monitoring of anticoagulation therapy; often the "referring" physician.
- *Cardiologist:* a specialist in finding, treating and preventing diseases of the heart and blood vessels; often referred to as the "plumber" of the heart.
- *Electrophysiologist:* a cardiologist who specializes in the electrical activity of the heart and in the diagnosis and treatment of heart rhythm disorders; often referred to as the "electrician" of the heart; (many but not all EPs perform catheter ablations such as radiofrequency or Cryo Pulmonary Vein Isolation procedures).
- *Cardiothoracic Surgeon:* performs surgery on the heart and blood vessels, such as the Cox-Maze and Mini-Maze surgeries; may have a cardiac specialty.

A TYPICAL 'SCENARIO' FOR A NEW A-FIB PATIENT

A typical scenario for a new A-Fib patient might be: Your General Practitioner (GP) arranges some basic tests to confirm your diagnosis, and then refers you to a Cardiologist. The Cardiologist puts you on multiple medications trying different drugs over the next six months to a year or more to see if any of these medications will stop or control your A-Fib. The drugs have limited success and the side effects make you miserable. After a year or more, your A-Fib continues, and your Cardiologist hasn't even mentioned the word "cure"!

Is this the best strategy for a new patient?

What's wrong with this scenario?

As you now know, A-Fib medications may not be very effective and often have unwanted side effects. And time is of the essence in treating A-Fib. The longer you wait, the more your A-Fib may "remodel" your heart, that is, change it physically and electrically.

Instead, it's probably better for you to see an Electrophysiologist (EP), a cardiologist who specializes in the electrical activity of the heart and in the diagnosis and treatment of heart rhythm disorders. You should seek an electrophysiologist who successfully restores A-Fib patients to normal sinus rhythm.

ORGANIZE YOUR RESEARCH

To find the right doctor to cure your A-Fib, start your research with a notebook and a file folder or binder. You need to organize the information you will be collecting: printouts of information from the internet, copies of documents from your local public library or medical center library, notes from phone calls, and answers to "interview" questions during doctor consultations. You may want to use a small tape or digital recorder during doctor appointments so that you can replay and review the conversation later (you will first ask the doctor's permission to record, of course).

Decide how and where you will keep your A-Fib research safe, yet easily accessible.

Understand Your Healthcare Coverage or Medical Policy

This may be a good time to mention the need to keep your medical coverage and/or healthcare policies handy. You will no doubt need to refer to these documents as you consider doctors, medical centers, and treatment options. You're sure to have questions such as "What is covered by my policy? What will be my out-or-pocket expense? What, if any, is the approval process? Can I direct bill or will I have to be reimbursed for my out-of-pocket expenses?"

It may be advantageous to ask a trusted family member or friend to help you maneuver through the maze of approvals, referrals, and plan coverage. (In addition, you may want to seek assistance through community-based or government-sponsored health insurance counseling and advocacy programs, as well as senior groups and other consumer advocacy organizations.)

COMPILE A LIST OF ELECTROPHYSIOLOGISTS

Beside personal referrals, widen your search for doctors through online search applications, such as the Heart Rhythm Society website feature, "Finding a

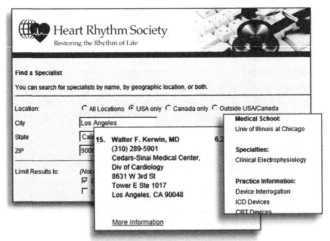

Visual 37: "Finding a Specialist" on the Heart Rhythm Society website.

Specialist" (refer to Appendix B for link).

It's easy to do. First, select your country of choice; if you choose the U.S., additional fields will appear with options to enter a city, state, zip code and/or radius. Enter data in one or more fields. To distinguish more experienced EPs in the PVI field, check the box for "Fellows of the HRS." A Fellow of the Heart Rhythm Society (FHRS) is an EP certified by the American Board of Internal Medicine (ABIM) in clinical cardiac electrophysiology (CCEP), has letters of support from current FHRS members, and has been vetted by the HRS Membership Committee. Lastly, click the "Locate" key.

Names of EPs will appear, each with contact information, medical school, specialties, and a Google map. To check whether they do Pulmonary Vein Isolations, click on "More Information." Under "Practice Information" it will list *AF Ablation* if they do Pulmonary Vein Isolation procedures.

Similar search services are provided by HealthGrades, Vitals.com, and the American Board of Medical Specialists (ABMS) Certification Matters.

Other Considerations

Many top EPs and leading medical centers are active in clinical research trials focused on developing new means of treating Atrial Fibrillation. For patients with particularly difficult or complex types of A-Fib, participation in clinical research trials opens up the possibility of treatment with emerging techniques not yet approved by the FDA.

If your type of A-Fib is difficult or complex, you may want to consult several of the leading electrophysiologists (outside of your geographic area). (The outcomes from Atrial Fibrillation ablations and other procedures are generally better in more experienced hands.)[227] Call or email to ask if you may send them your medicals records for review.

RESEARCH YOUR LIST

Research the credentials of prospective Electrophysiologists (EPs)—the names of their medical school and residency programs, board certifications, and patient ratings. Where and from whom did the doctor receive special training to treat A-Fib?

To find this information, consult the internet or your local public library or medical center library. The following resources will be helpful.

- The Official American Board of Medical Specialists (ABMS) Directory of Board Certified Medical Specialists;
- HealthGrades: an independent healthcare ratings organization provides physician's profile, education, patient reviews, awards & recognition, insurance accepted, hospital affiliations, malpractice or sanctions, locations.
- Online discussion groups and forums; read what other A-Fib patients have written about specific EPs.

Telephone and speak with the doctor's nurse or physician's assistant.

Armed with your list of EPs (and their contact information), telephone each doctor's office and speak with the doctor's nurse or physician's assistant.

After describing your type of A-Fib, ask questions about the doctor's practice (i.e., do they accept your health insurance), and treatment–related questions such as:

- How many patients with my type of A-Fib has the doctor treated?
- Of these patients, what percentage was treated with drug therapy only?
- What percentage was treated with catheter ablation procedures?
- What is the doctor's success rate? And how do you define "success"?
- Does the doctor refer patients for surgical procedures?

SET UP CONSULTATION APPOINTMENTS

With the information you have compiled, you should be able to narrow your list of doctors to a reasonable number. Rank order your list with the most promising choice first, followed by second, etc.

Next, set up in-office consultation appointments to "interview" your top three prospective electrophysiologists.

YOUR MEDICAL RECORDS

Obtain copies of your medical records, tests, and images.

Before meeting with any electrophysiologist, send each a copy of your medical records, tests results and any images/ X-rays.

You may ask, "Do I have a legal right to my medical records?" Yes—you have a right to view the originals and to obtain copies of your medical records.

Be aware that while the "information" belongs to you (the patient), the physical pieces of paper, X-ray film, etc. belong to the hospital or medical provider.[228] (In the U.S. this right is guaranteed by The Health Insurance Portability and Accountability Act of 1996 [HIPAA]. Your state laws may offer even greater rights than the federal act.)

Since you want to meet with several electrophysiologists to evaluate your treatment options, make or request several copies of your records. Allow sufficient time before your appointments for copying and shipping/delivery of your records. Expect to be charged for paper copies of medical reports. Electronic records may be provided to you on computer disks (CDs). Make copies for yourself or use an office supplies or copy center.

Your Personal A-Fib Medical Summary

Doctors appreciate knowledgeable, informed, and prepared patients. Each doctor will probably ask you much the same questions. For efficiency, you should prepare your answers and take along a copy (or send beforehand with your medical records).

As much as practical, provide your general health information such as allergies (especially to medicines), previous surgeries, other health events that resulted in hospitalizations, doctors you see regularly and why.

In their book, *Atrial Fibrillation: The Latest Management Strategies*,[229] Drs. Calkins and Berger suggest you prepare answers to several question before your appointment.

- What particular symptoms are bothering you?
- When did you first begin to experience these symptoms?

- Did you start taking any new vitamins, supplements, or prescription drugs before the onset of symptoms?
- Are these symptoms paroxysmal (occasional or intermittent, beginning and stopping on their own), or persistent (present all the time, or lasting at least a week at a time continuously)?
- On a scale of 1 to 5, with 1 being little or no bother and 5 being severely bothersome, how would you rate your symptoms?
- Is there anything that appears to worsen your symptoms?
- Is there anything that appears to lessen your symptoms?

Attach a copy of your "A-Fib Medical Summary" to your medical records for delivery beforehand or take a copy with you to your consultation.

PREPARING FOR YOUR CONSULTATIONS

We have prepared interview questions to help you collect information during each consultation appointment (see below). Don't worry about interviewing doctors. Remember---they will be "interviewing" you as well, to determine if they can help you. Don't limit yourself to our questions. Add your own questions.

In addition to medical topics, you should also assess the doctor's interpersonal style, demeanor and attentiveness. Is this someone you feel comfortable with and trust with your health care?

You may want to take along a trusted friend or family member as a personal advocate. They can accompany you to your appointment and press for coherent answers when needed, and verify you have answers to all the questions on your list. If needed, your personal advocate can question the doctor for you. In addition, consider using a tape or digital recorder to help you remember things. (Most doctors don't mind but always ask beforehand.)

After each interview, your personal advocate can help you evaluate the doctor's answers to your questions and discuss anything that's unclear to you. You may also want their opinion about your interaction and rapport with the doctor.

INTERVIEW QUESTIONS FOR ELECTROPHYSIOLOGISTS

This list of questions is designed to solicit information to help you select the best doctor for you and your type of A-Fib. After each question, we've included typical doctor responses and an analysis of what those responses may mean to you. Ask your doctor to draw pictures or use a model heart to explain answers, if that's helpful to you.

> 1. **What treatments do you recommend for dealing with or curing my type of A-Fib?**
>
> If the doctor only talks about different medications, you should probably thank them for their time and talk to other doctors on your list. Overall, drug therapies have poor success rates and don't address the progressive nature of Atrial Fibrillation.
>
> 2. **Do you perform Catheter Ablation procedures for my type of A-Fib? What type of procedures do you use or prefer?**
>
> RESPONSE #1: "I only work or prefer to work in the right atrium." Or, "I will eliminate the Atrial Flutter in your right atrium first."

These responses indicate a doctor may not have the experience or be comfortable working in the left atrium. Though it's more difficult to work in the left atrium, most A-Fib comes from the left atrium pulmonary veins. You may have Atrial Flutter in your right atrium along with your A-Fib, but it may well be triggered by the A-Fib coming from your left atrium.[230] If you hear this type of response, you should probably talk to other doctors on your list.

RESPONSE #2:   "We recommend catheter ablation of the AV Node and implanting a permanent pacemaker."

Though this used to be one of the most common treatments for A-Fib, you don't want to be burdened with a permanent pacemaker for the rest of your life when there are better options available.

Also, this procedure leaves you in A-Fib and dependent on medications for the rest of your life. Unless you have a Sinus Node problem and need a pacemaker, you should probably talk to other doctors on your list.

RESPONSE #3:   "We use Circumferential Ablation to eliminate A-Fib." Or "Segmental Ablation...." Or "Anatomically-Based Circumferential Ablation...." Or "Pulmonary Vein Antrum Isolation...."

Circumferential, Segmental, Anatomically-Based Circumferential (also referred to as Left Atrial Ablation or the Pappone technique) and Pulmonary Vein Antrum Isolation (PVAI) are refinements or different Pulmonary Vein Isolation procedure strategies. All offer you a good chance of being cured of your A-Fib. Circumferential is the most used technique.

RESPONSE #4:   "Besides RF catheters, we also use the CryoBalloon Catheter to isolate the Pulmonary Veins."

The CryoBalloon Catheter is a recent FDA-approved technology for A-Fib Ablation (approved December, 2010). In clinical trials, it was proven as effective, safer, and faster than the various types of RF ablation.

But, it is a relatively new method of ablation without a long-term track record of extensive data validating its effectiveness. However, anyone using the CryoBalloon Catheter is probably innovative, knowledgeable, and experienced in A-Fib ablation.

3. What is your success rate for my type of A-Fib? Does "success" mean I won't have to take any more antiarrhythmic drugs?

Major centers with extensive experience have a success rate of around 70%–85% for Paroxysmal (occasional) A-Fib, and a higher success rate if a second ablation is necessary. If their success rate is significantly less, you should probably look elsewhere.

Note: Some EPs consider a PVI a "success" if antiarrhythmic drugs which didn't work before now keep you in sinus rhythm.

However, Dr. Pierre Jais, from the French Bordeaux Group, defines success as restoring patients to normal sinus rhythm without dependence on any medications.[231]

4. *How long have you been performing catheter ablations for my type of A-Fib? How experienced are you with RF and/or Cryo? How many procedures do you perform a year?*

It's hard to quantify experience with specific numbers. But when doctors say they have done a total of 20 Pulmonary Vein Isolations, they are probably still in their "training" stage or have just passed their certification. And if a doctor only does a few PVIs a month, this may not be enough to maintain or develop ablation skills.

There are many electrophysiologists and several medical centers that have been doing Pulmonary Vein Isolation procedures for years and have done hundreds (or thousands) of PVIs.

5. *What kind of complications have your patients had after ablations?*

Every A-Fib doctor has had some complications when doing Pulmonary Vein Isolation procedures. A PVI is considered a lower risk procedure, for example, as compared to open heart surgery.[232] But it is not risk free. Possible complications include blood clots and stroke, PV Stenosis (post-op swelling of pulmonary vein openings which can restrict blood flow and lead to fatigue, flu-like symptoms, and pneumonia), and Cardiac Tamponade (pooling of fluid around the heart that can cause a drop in blood pressure).

Doctors and their office staff are usually very open about the complications they have had and can usually give you statistics. If they are not, you may want to look elsewhere for your doctor.

6. *What techniques or technologies do you use to increase the safety and effectiveness of your procedures? For example, how do you protect the esophagus from Atrial-Esophageal Fistula?*

A doctor's use of technology may improve their effectiveness compared to other doctors or medical centers.

For example: using an imaging system that gives 3–D images of the inside of the heart, of the position of the esophagus, and of catheter placement and pressure; using an energy source like the CryoBalloon catheter system to produce circular lesions around the pulmonary veins; using magnetic or robotic arms that aid in more precise placements of lesions or ablations.

When you ask how the doctor protects the esophagus, you should hear answers like:

RESPONSE 1:   "We use low power at the back of the heart."
RESPONSE 2:   "We use a temperature probe in the esophagus to make sure it doesn't get too hot."
RESPONSE 3:   "We use barium paste in the esophagus so that we can see where it is when we make ablations and don't make ablations near the esophagus."

RESPONSE 4: "We give Proton Pump Inhibitors like Nexium for two–three weeks after an ablation to protect the esophagus."

If you don't get answers like these, especially about taking Proton Pump Inhibitors after an ablation, it might be wise to consider other doctors.

7. Do you ever refer your patients for a Cox-Maze or Mini-Maze surgery?

Some A-Fib patients might be better served by a Cox-Maze or Mini-Maze surgery. For example, someone who needs heart surgery for another problem might well combine that surgery with a Cox-Maze operation. Someone who can't tolerate Coumadin or other blood thinners might be better served by a Mini-Maze surgery. Most Mini-Maze surgeries are the result of referrals by electrophysiologists.

If a doctor doesn't normally refer patients for Cox-Maze surgeries, this isn't necessarily a reason for rejection. They may be concerned about a loss of quality control if they send patients to someone who's not a specialist in heart rhythm problems.

8. (For female patients) What is the extent of your training specifically related to women's heart health?

Women tend to have different symptoms of heart disease than men, in part because their bodies respond differently to risk factors such as high blood pressure. Cardiologists who specialize in women are more common than ever. Medical centers now have clinics devoted to women's heart health. Women with A-Fib may want to seek out a specialist who is up-to-date in this field of research.

Before your consultation is over, briefly repeat back to the doctor what was said to make sure you have understood and your notes are accurate.

Did you get through all your questions? If not, let your doctor know you need more time. Some doctors will offer to call you after office hours to continue your conversation. Or perhaps you can speak to a nurse or physician assistant instead.

INTERVIEW QUESTIONS FOR CARDIAC SURGEONS

Have you been referred to a surgeon? Are you considering a surgical option to cure your A-Fib? If so, you need to discuss some very specific issues. (As with the questions for EPs, we've inserted information to help you assess their answers.)

Remember: ask your doctor to draw pictures or use a model heart if that might help to explain something.

1. Preliminary questions for surgeons treating Atrial Fibrillation:

  a. What treatment do you recommend for dealing with or curing my type of A-Fib?

  b. What is your success rate for my type of A-Fib? Does "success" mean I won't have to take any more antiarrhythmic drugs?

  c. How long have you been performing surgery for my type of A-Fib?

  d. How many surgeries of this type do you perform a year?

2. If I choose a Cox-Maze or Mini-Maze surgery:

  a. *How will you access the heart? Open-chest? If key-hole incisions, how many incisions will the procedure require?*

      b.   *(Cox-Maze): Will I need to be on heart/lung bypass? (Mini-Maze): Will you deflate and inflate my lungs? What are the associated risks?*

      c.   *What is my risk of stroke during or after the surgery?*

      d.   *How long is the recovery period, in and out of the hospital?*

3. **Would a catheter ablation fix my A-Fib without the added risk of heart surgery? A Pulmonary Vein Isolation, for example?**

A Cox-Maze or Mini-Maze operation is still cardiac surgery with the associated risks. It's important to discuss catheter ablation as an alternative to surgery.

4. **If I choose a Mini-Maze surgery, how extensive are the ablation lines to the Left Atrium?**

      a.   *Are these ablation lines limited to the pulmonary veins?*

      b.   *What if A-Fib signals are coming from other areas of my heart?*

      c.   *Is this amount of ablation lines and scarring necessary to fix my type of A-Fib?*

      d.   *Will this scarring permanently affect other heart functions?*

The newer versions of the Mini-Maze (i.e., the Totally Thoracoscopic (TT) Maze, the Five-Box Thoracoscopic Maze, and the Dallas Extended Lesion Set) include ablation and scarring of the left atrium. This burning and scarring can cause problems with circulation, nerve signal pathways, heart muscle fibers and transport function, etc. Discuss these possible complications with the surgeon. (Have the surgeon explain or point out on a model heart each scar they will make, and why each burn is necessary for your heart.)

5. **Will you staple shut or close off the Left Atrial Appendage (LAA)? Is this necessary if you expect me to be A-Fib free after the surgery?**

The Left Atrial Appendage acts as a "release valve" for the atrium and performs other functions. Some question the need to close off the LAA if the patient will be A-Fib free after the surgery.

      a.   *If the LAA will be closed off, what technique will you use (i.e., suture, stapler or AtriClip)?*

      b.   *How do you know if you have successfully closed off the entire LAA?*

A recent study found both suture and stapler methods had extraordinarily low success rates for closing off the LAA. Use of the newer AtriClip looks more promising.

6. **(For Atrial Flutter patients) If I have a Mini-Maze surgery for my A-Fib, how will my Atrial Flutter be handled?**

Current Mini-Maze surgeries do not address Atrial Flutter. The standard treatment for Flutter is catheter ablation.

EVALUATE EACH INTERVIEW

After each appointment, first reflect on your rapport with the doctor. Consider how you felt during the meeting.

- Was the doctor attentive? Did you feel relaxed? Or did you feel rushed? Or were you intimidated or overpowered by the doctor?
- Did the doctor listen to you? Were your questions welcomed? Or was the doctor annoyed or dismissive? Did he or she seem to trust your own instincts and perceptions of your health?
- Just as important, did the doctor answer in easy-to-understand terms? Were models or drawings used to help explain procedural or surgical steps or goals to you?
- Did you feel a collaboration developing? Do you now feel confident in and trust this doctor?
- How were you treated by the office personnel? Was the staff attentive and helpful? Were they courteous? Did they seem to welcome your questions?

Next, compare the doctor's answers to our analysis of possible answers. As needed, discuss your notes with your personal advocate. You may find their observations insightful. If you need further explanation of terms the doctor used, refer to our Glossary of Medical Terms.

Rank this doctor compared to other doctors you have interviewed.

Make note of your impression of this doctor. (Keep in mind you might want to consult this doctor later for a second opinion.) Store your notes with your other research papers.

MAKING YOUR DECISION

When you consider each of your doctor interviews, did one doctor stand out as your first choice? Or, are you uncertain? Or are you dissatisfied with the lot? If so, meet with one or more of the other doctors on your list and repeat the evaluation process.

Be courageous, be persistent. Don't decide on an electrophysiologist or surgeon until you get answers to all your questions. Make sure you've discussed all your treatment options, and you have a good rapport with the doctor.

A BETTER 'SCENARIO' FOR THE NEW A-FIB PATIENT

A better scenario for a new A-Fib patient might be: Your GP recommends several electrophysiologists. You check the A-Fib Discussion Groups on the internet for additional recommendations. You search for EPs using online physician referral sites like HRS. You compile a list.

You research each doctor on your list, on the internet and with other A-Fib patients. You read about their education, training, experience, and reputation. You call each medical office and question the doctor's nurse or physician's assistant. Then, you rank order the EPs or surgeons and schedule a "consultation" appointment with your top choices. You send copies of your medical records beforehand.

During each in office "interview", you ask your prepared questions and note their responses. In addition, you consider the doctor's manner, viewpoints, and personality.

Afterwards, you reflect on your rapport with each doctor and evaluate the doctor's answers. You ponder, "Does this doctor understand how A-Fib affects me? Is this someone who can solve my problem? Is this someone who inspires my confidence, whom I can trust?" If not, or if you are uncertain, you meet with one or more of the other doctors on your list until you find the right one for you.

The end result of this scenario is finding the right doctor for you, for your type of A-Fib and for your desired outcome. You have become your own best patient advocate.

SUMMARY

As an Atrial Fibrillation patient, you must take responsibility for finding your cure. Continue to educate yourself (as you are now by reading this book). Seek the advice of current and former A-Fib patients. Consult several doctors, as necessary, to find the right doctor and/or medical center for you.

If you decide to consider both ablation and surgical options, it's essential to understand factors unique to each treatment. Prepare for each consultation with the appropriate list of questions. Afterwards, evaluate the answers from each doctor and note your rapport with each before making your decision.

❖

At this point, you may be curious about other A-Fib patients who have searched for an A-Fib cure. In the next chapter you'll find real stories related by A-Fib patients themselves. You'll read stories shared by both men and women from various age groups, from different parts of the world, and with various types of A-Fib who made a range of treatment choices. You'll read about their "lessons learned" and their advice to you. You'll read how many are now living a life free of the burden A-Fib.

May the next chapter give you hope and inspire you to find your own A-Fib cure.

❖

CHAPTER ELEVEN

Personal Stories of Hope, Courage, and Lessons Learned

Others have been where you are right now. In their own words, these fellow A-Fib patients offer their stories...to encourage you, to advise you, to bolster your resolve, and to offer you hope of a life free of A-Fib—including lessons learned the hard way—through first-hand experience.

EDITOR'S COMMENTS OFFER INSIGHTS

Study the "Editorial Comments" which follow each patient's story. You'll find pertinent medical information and explanations to help you understand the problems or conditions described and insight as to their significance.

CROSS-REFERENCED BY THEME AND TOPIC

While all the stories are inspiring, feel free to read just the stories that interest you. Here's a list of themes and topics cross-referenced to story number:

- Causes: holiday heart [2, 3], binge drinking [13], and heredity [7]
- Anxiety and stress [2, 3, 4, 12]
- Heart attack, stroke and risks of clots [7, 9, 10, 15]
- Drug Therapy [1, 5, 6, 10, 12, 15), Pill-In-Pocket [2, 8], and side effects [11, 13, 14]
- Cardioversion [2, 13]
- Pulmonary Vein Isolation [1, 2, 3, 6, 8, 13], and Cryoablation [9, 12]
- Maze and Mini-Maze Surgeries [5, 7, 11, 14] and LAA closure/AtriClip [11]
- AV Node Ablation/Pacemaker [7, 16]
- Watchman device [10, 15, 16]

INTRODUCTION TO PERSONAL STORIES

1. *Michele: Cured After 30 Years But Had to Get Mad—at Her A-Fib Heart and Her Doctor*

Michele's story takes a turn toward a cure when she got mad, "... so mad at my heart and at my cardiologist, who basically spent five minutes with me once a year and said my life was as good as it was going to get."

2. *Max: From Finland to China to France A-Fib Was Devastating, Days Start With 7 AM Attack*

Max is a lawyer working in China (PRC). He describes how his first A-Fib episode was thought to be "holiday heart." But his A-Fib escalated, and each day began with a regular 7 AM attack. He describes how A-Fib caused him to be obnoxious towards his wife and colleagues and how he became desperate for a cure.

3. *Jay: For This Father of Four Youngsters, A-Fib Began at Age 25!*

Jay, a young father of four little ones, relates how anxiety was his greatest challenge. After a successful second "touch up" ablation, it's now more than four years later. Jay's still free of A-Fib and counting his blessings.

4. *Kelly: The Spouse's Prospective, a Young Wife and Mother Copes With Husband's A-Fib*

Kelly married Jay just months after he had his first A-Fib attack. Today, ten years later, Kelly describes what it was like raising four children while trying to cope with her husband's Atrial Fibrillation.

5. *Sheri: A Life on Meds Wasn't Good Enough—Selects a Minimally Invasive Cox-Maze IV*

Sheri didn't want a life on medication. While still in the hospital and dissatisfied with her doctor's lack of alternatives, she researched her options and found her way to a life free of both medications and her A-Fib.

6. *Warren: A-Fib Burden Lifted After Consulting a New Cardiologist Down Under*

Aussie Warren's first cardiologist was critical of catheter ablation. When the burden of his A-Fib worsened, Warren did his own online research and decided to change cardiologists. He got the ablations he needed, and now for the first time since 1998 he's A-Fib free.

7. *Roger: In 2000 Chooses a Full Surgical Cox-Maze (Open Chest); Three Generations with A-Fib*

Roger, a former U.S. Marine, watched his father cope with Atrial Fibrillation and then developed it himself. In 2000, at age 65, he had a full surgical Cox-Maze (open chest). In hindsight, he thinks he may have rushed into that decision to avoid going on Coumadin. Since then, cardio health challenges continued to unfold for him, including a daughter developing A-Fib.

8. *Joan: First in Denial, then Pill-in-the-Pocket Served Her Well For Years*

Joan's A-Fib crept slowly into her life, her second episode not occurring until four years after the first. But each year that followed had an increasing number of episodes until a new cardiologist recommended a treatment change.

9. *Ken: Heart Attacks & Bypass Surgeries, But A-Fib Free After a CryoBalloon Ablation*

Ken developed A-Fib in 1992 post-op in the Intensive Care Unit (ICU) following quad bypass heart surgery. Controlled with medication for 15 years, a second bypass surgery ignited his A-Fib once again. Finally, in 2010, he found his cure through a CryoBalloon ablation procedure.

10. *Tom: With 'Silent' A-Fib Decides on Watchman Device to Ditch the Drugs*

Tom has Silent A-Fib (A-Fib with few noticeable symptoms) and had been on Coumadin for six years to address the associated risk of clots and an A-Fib stroke. Then, out of the blue, a phone call offered him an alternative to the meds and monthly blood tests.

11. *Joy: Annoying A-Fib Symptoms Worsen & Turn Critical With Threat of Sick Sinus Syndrome*

For years Joy's A-Fib symptoms were mostly annoying. In 2010 they worsened into near-fainting episodes. Fear of an A-Fib episode overshadowed activities she once enjoyed with her teenage daughter. On the verge of developing sick sinus syndrome, she had a decision to make.

12. *Terry: Misdiagnosed as Anxiety, Later Found A-Fib Cure Through a Clinical Trial*

Terry was seeing a therapist because he thought his "attacks" were caused by anxiety; after his A-Fib diagnosis, many drug therapies followed. His cure came in 2007 from a clinical trial for CryoBalloon ablation.

13. *Kris: Binge Drinking Leads To Chronic A-Fib, Amiodarone Damages Eyesight*

Kris was admitted for double pneumonia when they discovered the A-Fib. She tells how her A-Fib was brought on by a combination of alcohol, stress, bacterial pneumonia and over-the-counter cold medications.

14. *Daniel: A-Fib Returns after 8 years, Opts for Totally Thoracoscopic (TT) Mini-Maze*

Daniel thought he had whipped his A-Fib, so after a year he stopped his meds. Eight years later it returned, along with Atrial Flutter this time. Meds were successful, but with unacceptable side effects. He opted for a Totally Thoracoscopic (TT) Mini-Maze operation.

15. *David: Two Hematomas + Hemorrhagic Stroke = Worries About Blood Clots*

David had a worst case scenario as an A-Fib patient. While on Coumadin, he had a hemorrhagic stroke (bleeding in the brain). He recovered and discovered, like many A-Fib patients, that he could not tolerate blood thinners. But how was he to combat the risk of blood clots and A-Fib stroke without the aid of blood thinners?

16. *Emmett: 40-Year Battle with A-Fib Includes AV Node Ablation With Pacemaker*

Emmett was with the L.A. City Fire Dept. for 27 years. His 40-year story with A-Fib demonstrates, first hand, the recent evolution in the treatment of Atrial Fibrillation including PVIs, an AV Node ablation and, most recently, the Watchman procedure.

❖

Cured After 30 Years But Had to Get Mad—at Her A-Fib Heart and Her Doctor

Michele's story takes a turn toward a cure when she got mad, "... so mad at my heart and at my cardiologist, who basically spent five minutes with me once a year and said my life was as good as it was going to get."

I WAS DIAGNOSED with A-Fib 30 years ago, but I don't really know how long I'd had it as I was mostly asymptomatic unless exercising during air pollution episodes ("red alert" days) and when sick. I was in A-Fib 24/7 all that time. We have no idea why I went into A-Fib.

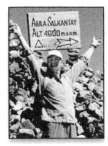

Michele Straube
Salt Lake City, Utah, USA

HIT OR MISS WITH MEDS AND CARDIOLOGISTS

My experiences with cardiologists were hit and miss. Early on I was told that they had never seen someone so young with A-Fib (at the time, I was in my mid 20s), and some told me the best they could do was medicate me so I could walk from the bed to the window and back. *I changed doctors.*

Others wanted to give me all kinds of meds, which I researched and refused to take. I had one cardioversion which took for a few days; I didn't try another. In the end, I took digoxin for years (which did nothing much except minimal rate control) and then calcium channel blockers for about ten years (which actually controlled my rate so that I could exercise moderately). I refused to take Coumadin/warfarin (blood thinners) and took aspirin instead.

DECIDING TO HAVE AN ABLATION

In the fall of 2009, I decided to have an ablation. I had gone on a trek in Peru the summer before and it about killed me. I got so mad at my heart and at my cardiologist (who basically spent five minutes with me once a year and said my life was as good as it was going to get). I decided at the top of the highest pass in Peru to change cardiologists when I got back home.

> ❖ *"I got so mad at my heart and at my cardiologist... I decided at the top of the highest pass in Peru to change cardiologists when I got back home."*
>
> Michele Straube

In researching doctors in my area, I learned that ablation procedures have greatly advanced in the past few years. I also knew that my risk of stroke was increasing with age and with the length of time I was in A-Fib (meaning I'd probably have to switch to Coumadin in the next five years or so).

ABLATION BY DR. MARROUCHE

So, I went to a new doctor, Dr. Nassir Marrouche at the University of Utah's Cardiovascular Center in Salt Lake City. To determine whether you are a good candidate for ablation, Dr. Marrouche includes a cardiac MRI to identify areas and extent of fibrosis in your heart (i.e., too much fibrosis = not so good a candidate). After doing my cardiac MRI, he felt I was a good candidate for an ablation.

Given my age and my risks with the history of A-Fib, I was willing to take this step for the possibility of no more meds in the future and an improved quality of life. The ablation was done by Dr. Marrouche in November 2009.

SUCCESS! IN NORMAL SINUS RHYTHM

I am now more than 2 years post-ablation, free of A-Fib and feeling terrific. I am still (knock on wood) in NSR (normal sinus rhythm). Most importantly, my quality of life is SO IMPROVED.

I can ride a bike again for the first time in 20 years or so (going downhill is so much fun, going uphill is still work). I'm training for a local A-Fib Awareness 5K; I can already jog about half the distance (I hadn't run for over five years before the ablation). I'm taking Zumba classes and adult ballet lessons and loving every sore muscle.

> ❖ *"I can climb a flight of stairs without wheezing; I don't collapse on the couch at 6 PM, etc."*
>
> Michele Straube

I have much more energy and stamina. I make it through the work day without having to sit down and rest all the time. I can exercise at levels I can't remember since my teenage years (30–35 years ago). All the side effects of the heart medications are GONE, meaning I feel great every day.

The other major quality of life improvement is no more dizziness. I can now join in on any activity or family event knowing that I will not get faint or have to sit on the sidelines due to fatigue. I can easily stand listening to my daughter's *School of Rock* gigs for an hour or more (we used to always bring a chair for me to be slightly dizzy in); I can climb a flight of stairs without wheezing; I don't collapse on the couch at 6 PM, etc.

CROSS THE HEART OF THE ALPS FOR A-FIB AWARENESS

Just walking uphill fast is a miracle, but now I can do that and talk at the same time, or carry a 20-lb backpack and make it up without wheezing or dizziness.

I revived a dream to walk the Via Alpina (approx. 1500 miles up and over the Alps through eight countries). In the summer of 2011, my husband and I walked the first leg of the trek, and will walk again each summer crossing the Alps in three or four trips.

Trekking in the Alps was fantastic. I trained tons before we went, but I was still surprised with how hard it was. Even though my aerobic capacity keeps improving the longer I am out of A-Fib, I'm not sure I'll ever have the stamina of people my age who have been heart healthy and physically active all along. Ah well, I'm definitely not complaining. I no longer have to choose the hike based on distance or elevation gain—going 'slowly slowly'. It is so exciting to be able to go hiking in the surrounding mountains; I am crossing new attained goals off my list every weekend.

Life is so good!

LESSONS LEARNED

I wish the CARMA's (Comprehensive Arrhythmia Research & Management Center, Un. of Utah) MRI-screening and ranking methodology had existed earlier. I would not have spent ten years incorrectly thinking an ablation would not work for me (it would and did work for me). It's vital to find out what's going on inside your heart (through an MRI) before you and your doctor make decisions about what's possible and what's not.

My advice to those with A-Fib:

- Go to an electrophysiologist A-Fib expert right away, one with a high success rate at getting patients back into normal rhythm — you deserve nothing less.
- Do not take "this is as good as it gets" as an answer— do your own research about what's possible and take a co-leadership role with your doctor.
- Keep doing as much as you possibly can while in A-Fib (e.g., exercise) without jeopardizing your health. I am convinced that a strong heart muscle can only benefit you, especially if and when you get back into normal rhythm.

The earlier cardiologists treated me like an 80-year-old A-Fib patient, assuming that reducing the risk of stroke was the only "treatment" needed or appropriate. I'm glad I had lofty exercise goals while in A-Fib (e.g., I want to continue hiking mountains) and that my more recent cardiologists helped me maintain the highest quality of life possible.

My ablation miracle continues.

Michele Straube
Salt Lake City, Utah, USA

Editorial Comments:

Michele's cardiologist, Dr. Nassir Marrouche is making significant advances in the treatment of A-Fib through his research on Atrial Fibrosis (fiber-like structural changes to the normally smooth walls of the heart).

After 30 years in A-Fib, it's surprising Michele's heart wasn't more fibrotic. With only 18% fibrotic tissue, Dr. Marrouche placed her in what he calls "Utah 2" (5%–20% scarring/fibrosis in the heart). Over 35% fibrosis—"Utah 4" he considers poor candidates for a Pulmonary Vein Isolation procedure.

This research is important as Fibrosis increases your risk of A-Fib stroke, and is a factor in the successful outcome of catheter ablations.

Her story also demonstrates the importance of working with the right doctor for your symptoms, and your attitude about your illness. Has your doctor offered you treatment options besides drug therapy? Is your doctor current on A-Fib research and non-pharmaceutical options? If not, you may want to talk with other doctors.

That's what Michele did. She found a cardiologist who did more than talk with her for five minutes once a year, who did more than just say a life on drugs "was as good as it was going to get." She got fed up with her illness and its impact on her quality of life. She did her homework and found a new cardiologist, one who offered her an ablation procedure to fix her Atrial Fibrillation. Her choices lead to her cure. These days she can climb the Alps—A-Fib-free. See Michele's blog: Into the Heart of the Alps.

❖

From Finland to China to France A-Fib Was Devastating, Days Start with 7am Attack

Max is a lawyer working in China (PRC). He describes how his first A-Fib episode was thought to be just "holiday heart." But his A-Fib escalated, and each day began with a regular 7 AM attack. He describes how A-Fib caused him to be obnoxious towards his wife and colleagues and how he became desperate for a cure.

I AM A FINNISH lawyer working in Shanghai, People's Republic of China (PRC) since 1996. My work is rather stressful and from time to time, very hectic, but I love it. I mostly deal with corporate and commercial law but also with project financing.

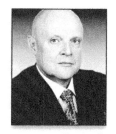

Max Jussila
Shanghai, China

FIRST A-FIB ATTACKS

I experienced my first event of Atrial Fibrillation in 2003, at age 47, on a beautiful summer morning in Finland. I was on a holiday from China. During the previous night some friends and I had had BBQ with quite excessive drinking. The doctors at the ER immediately called it a "weekend heart" or "holiday heart;" and since it converted by itself in just a few minutes after an ECG had been taken and the diagnosis made, they just sent me home. I was not given any medication at that time nor was I prescribed anything to take on a permanent basis.

The second incident appeared more than half a year later, also in Finland, on winter holiday; but this time I hadn't had any alcohol to drink. I went to the ER. And while I was waiting (EKG was already taken), the A-Fib converted by itself after maybe a half-hour again. I made an appointment with a cardiologist. He did the routine tests, lipid panel, heart echo, and stress test on a bike and told me my heart was in excellent condition. But based on the EKG, I unfortunately had paroxysmal Atrial Fibrillation.

> ❖ *"He also told me that many people have it (A-Fib) and it is not dangerous."*
>
> Max Jussila

He also told me that many people have it, and it is not dangerous. [TO THE CONTRARY, A-FIB IS DANGEROUS AND CAN CAUSE STROKE AND OTHER HEART PROBLEMS.] I started metoprolol beta blockers and tried to forget the whole thing. My A-Fib stayed away for almost a year. I don't believe that metoprolol had anything to do with the benign outcome. We just don't know how often the incidents occur, and it's really different from person to person.

DEVASTATING EFFECTS OF A-FIB

After that peaceful year it was all down-hill for me. I started having A-Fib attacks, PACs (premature atrial contractions) and PVCs (premature ventricle contractions) more and more often and had to be cardioverted electronically a few times.

The Christmas of 2007 and early 2008 until the end of the year was absolutely the worst time that I have ever experienced. I was in A-Fib on and off, and nothing seemed to help. I had Rythmol as a Pill-in-the-Pocket (PIP). It usually helped to convert the A-Fib; but after each incident and having taken Rhythmol, I was totally exhausted. And I had started getting A-Fibs every morning around 7 o'clock, regularly. The good thing was that they very often converted while taking a shower or on my way to the foreign clinic in Shanghai.

I was, however, constantly working. And I have to say that I have never been mentally so incapable and in plain words "stupid" as I was during that time. My memory was gone, my speech was gone (I speak five languages), and even the simplest work-related problems seemed impossible for me to handle, let alone solve.

> ❖ "...but mentally I was reduced to a six-year-old child with constant tantrums."
>
> Max Jussila

I had become totally obnoxious towards my wife and colleagues, and I was absolutely desperate. I was only 52 years old; I should have been at the peak of my professional skills and capabilities at that age, but mentally I was reduced to a six–year-old child with constant tantrums.

I understood that I had to do something about my situation.

DECIDING TO GO TO BORDEAUX

I started surfing the Internet and found Steve Ryan's website (A-Fib.com). What a day! I studied everything very carefully and meticulously, discussed with my wife and with my Chinese cardiologist (a very nice chap). Since he supported my decision to have a catheter ablation (mind you, I'd have had it done even if he'd been against the whole thing!), I wrote to Bordeaux in August 2008. I was given a time nine months later.

> ❖ "I started surfing the Internet and... I studied everything very carefully and meticulously."
>
> Max Jussila

Since I had A-Fibs now on a daily basis and was seriously frightened that the Atrial Fibrillation would become persistent, I wrote to Bordeaux again asking for an earlier appointment. The response was positive, and I was scheduled for a catheter ablation on 19 January 2009.

FIRST ABLATION

I first flew to Finland to see my 90–year-old Mother (who is in persistent A-Fib), and had a TEE (trans-esophageal echocardiogram) done in Helsinki. It took about 15 minutes and was not at all unpleasant: the doctor sprayed "something" (novocaine?) into my throat and inserted the catheter, checked, found nothing, and it was over.

I then flew to Paris, took the bullet train to Bordeaux, and stayed two nights at the Holiday Inn near the heart clinic of Hôpital Haut Lévêque—Bordeaux Pessac. I went to downtown Bordeaux to see the city which was an experience per se.

On Monday the 19th I went to the hospital around 1 PM. The welcome was very warm and professional, most of the nurses understood English and my rusty French, my private room was very nice, food was good, and everything made me feel confident. About 1:30 PM a nurse rushed in and gave me a bottle of Betadine solution (bacteria-killing shower soap), and told me to take a pre-operational shower. She was going to come and shave my groin after fifteen minutes, and I was supposed to be taken to the OR to have the ablation done.

The ablation was actually scheduled for the next day, Tuesday, but why not? I did as I was told, and very quickly I was down in the OR where a very pleasant and soft-spoken (and gorgeous) Dr. Mélèze Hocini introduced herself, asked how I felt, and told me that she'll perform the ablation.

I was given local anaesthesia on my right groin, and Dr. Hocini started. During the ablation I received something for pain. The pain was not unbearable but might have been unpleasant without the medication. So, I was conscious all the time. And Dr. Hocini told me every now and then what she was doing which was very interesting.

> ❖ "So, I was conscious all the time. And Dr. Hocini told me every now and then what she was doing which was very interesting."
>
> Max Jussila

Dr. Pierre Jaïs popped in after a while to lead a catheter through the septal wall in my heart. Dr. Hocini finished after 6.5 hours having isolated all the pulmonary veins and ablated the cavotricuspid isthmus with complete linear block. It was 8 PM, and she was totally finished, I could see that. A more than 12–hour working day for her, which I understand is not anything exceptional. I just have to admire these wonderful people!

The post-ablation stay of five days and the check-up next Monday went fine, nothing in the stress test or otherwise. I cannot say that I had any chest pain really, just a little bit uncomfortable feeling. But the bed in OR had been quite uncomfortable, and I had been lying on it for 6.5 hours and could certainly feel that.

I was given Nexium 40 mg to prevent esophageal fistula, and Coumadin to prevent blood clots. During my stay at the hospital I watched history documentaries on my computer from CDs I had brought with me.

A-FLUTTER POST ABLATION

I flew home to Shanghai, but problems started a couple of weeks after the ablation. I had two subsequent A-Fibs, which converted by themselves.

But then a Flutter began. It was electrocardioverted five times but persisted. I had to fly to Beijing to negotiations and was in Flutter with a heart rate of 108. The Flutter lasted for a couple of weeks despite taking flecainide, and then suddenly converted into normal sinus rhythm at a wedding we attended on 9 March. I couldn't believe the feeling!

> ❖ "I was given Nexium 40 mg to prevent esophageal fistula, and Coumadin to prevent blood clots."
>
> Max Jussila

SECOND ABLATION

I had already been in contact with Dr. Hocini who agreed to a second ablation. The second one took place on 30 March 2009. The experience was exactly like the first one: I was very well and professionally treated, and I really felt confident that I was in very good hands.

Now two doctors were working on me, Dr. Hocini and Dr. Michel Haïssaguerre. It took them another 6.5 hours to ablate. This is how the doctors described the procedure:

"The PVs remained isolated. Burst atrial pacing induced several AT (atrial tachycardia) mainly with a focal mechanism and one rotating around the mitral annulus. A mitral isthmus line was performed which resulted in transformation of the tachycardia to A-Fib. That A-Fib terminated after targeting all fractionated and complex sites in the right and left atria.

Finally termination of A-Fib was obtained during ablation at the right atrial appendage. Following this, atrial pacing demonstrated a complete linear block at the LA roof, mitral isthmus and cavotricuspid isthmus."

> ❖ *"I was told my case was really difficult...as evidenced by their ablation of the right atrial appendage, which I understand is seldom done."*
>
> Max Jussila

I was told my case was really difficult (I'm not bragging) as evidenced by their ablation of the right atrial appendage, which I understand is seldom done. Post-ablation time at the hospital (three days) went without any incidents, and I returned to Shanghai.

Maybe it was due to the skills of the doctors, but after those two ablations I had no chest pain, no bruises in my groin, nothing to make me feel uncomfortable. I also think that it's a good thing not to be sedated during the procedure, because that way you are aware of what is happening around you and can even interact with the doctors.

The only "uncomfortable" thing was the amount of fluids that were pumped into me, so I had to ask for a bottle to urinate in three times during the procedure.

FINALLY FEELING CURED

I kept a diary of my "feelings", and I have to say that this time I actually really felt that I was cured. In the early weeks of April 2009, I could feel some extra systoles (an irregularity in the heart rhythm), but nothing really bad. I experienced one strange night by the end of April when I had really bad nightmares, but I have no idea whether they were heart-related or not, and I guess not.

> ❖ *"I kept a diary of my "feelings" and I have to say that this time I actually really felt that I was cured."*
>
> Max Jussila

I had the first post-ablation 24–hour Holter monitor study done on 14 May with just three supraventricular ectopics (heartbeat signals that come from any region of the heart that ordinarily should not produce them), nothing else.

After all that I have experienced I'm quite sure I know what my heart is doing, whether it's in A-Fib, Flutter or something else!

> ❖ *"I was given my life back, literally, by the extremely skillful doctors in Bordeaux."*
>
> Max Jussila

Since the second ablation I've felt nothing really bad except some occasional extra beats (a 24–hour Holter showed only four supraventricular and two ventricular ectopics). I am 54 years old now, and my heart rate is a steady 70 and my BP is 120/75 (this morning). I was given my life back, literally, by the extremely skillful doctors in Bordeaux.

I have started Chinese Kung Fu, san da–style which is practiced by the Chinese Army Special Forces (extremely good for muscles and joints), I exercise on my bike watching CNN news broadcasts half an hour twice per day, do some weight-lifting and swimming, and will most likely take up diving again. I cannot believe what a wreck I was before these two catheter ablations!

I am very grateful to Steve for his wonderfully informative website, A-Fib.com. I am an A-Fib.com Support Volunteer in China and am happy to help others get through the ordeal of A-Fib.

Whatever happens later on, I will be eternally grateful to the wonderful doctors in Bordeaux (especially Dr. Hocini who is a straight shooter as well). They are refining their methods every day; and I am sure they will reach more and more people, that the results will become even better everywhere in the world.

> ❖ *"The doctors who see medication as a solution commit serious negligence...."*
>
> Max Jussila

LESSONS LEARNED

To all those who suffer from this terrible condition called Atrial Fibrillation: do not listen to your doctor if he/she suggests medication as a long-term solution! Medication is a very short-term and temporary phase to keep you somewhat functional for a short period of time BEFORE catheter ablation.

The doctors who see medication as a solution commit serious negligence and are ignorant of the terrible nature and consequences of Atrial Fibrillation.

Max Jussila
Shanghai, China

Editorial Comments:

As Max recounts, living in A-Fib can have devastating and life-changing psychological effects. A-Fib affects not only you but also impacts your family, friends and work colleagues. Consider talking one-on-one with them. They probably know little or nothing about Atrial Fibrillation. Be honest and up front. Share your symptoms, how A-Fib makes you feel, and how it affects your daily activities and responsibilities. Answer their questions.

In 2009, Max found his A-Fib cure through PVIs performed in Bordeaux, France (same as the author in 1998). The French Bordeaux group invented Pulmonary Vein Isolation and is still considered by many to be the best in the world. But it's not necessary to go to France to be cured of A-Fib. Thousands of A-Fib centers worldwide now perform successful Pulmonary Vein Isolation (PVI) procedures.

❖

For This Father of Four Youngsters, A-Fib Began at Age 25

Jay, a young father of four little ones, relates how anxiety was his greatest challenge. After a successful second "touch up" ablation, it's now more than three years later. Jay's still free of A-Fib and counting his blessings.

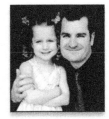

MY A-FIB STORY begins at age 25 (before marriage and kids). As with many people, my attack began suddenly and without warning. My A-Fib presented with a very rapid heartbeat; so it was a rather scary event, especially for a 25 year old. I had been at a dinner party and drank some wine. The doctors in the ER pronounced it "holiday heart" and informed me that I would likely never deal with this again. I stayed in A-Fib for six days that first time. My heart eventually converted on its own with medication, after which time

Jay Teresi and daughter
Ayla, Atlanta, GA, USA

the doctors ended the medication; and I mostly forgot about the whole episode.

My second experience with A-Fib occurred two years later during a round of golf (I was 27 years old). The doctors felt that I was dehydrated, and again announced that I would likely never experience this again. My heart converted after 24 hours with medication. (This time I was admitted to the intensive care unit overnight, so needless to say that got my attention. I have since learned that this was an overreaction on the hospital's part.)

Although I was told to forget about A-Fib, I found that I could not. I made many lifestyle changes, quit drinking altogether, began exercising, and eating healthier.

Life moved on, and I was promoted to Austin, TX and moved there from California. After a year I began to feel better and not worry so much; then the third episode occurred. This time, however, things were different. The doctors in TX were very aggressive; and after two hours of no response to medications in the ER, they cardioverted me on the spot in the ER (to this point I never even knew that was an option, had never heard of cardioversion).

FIRST ABLATION AND A-FIB FREE

I was placed on medication to regulate rhythm. For whatever reason, I had many side effects. It was a tough five months. My cardiologist sent me to an EP doctor who talked to me about ablation. I didn't even know that was possible. I was very excited about being free of A-Fib, since I had allowed it to start limiting my activities (quit camping, hard exercise, and stopped enjoying most activities I found pleasurable before the episodes). I had my first ablation in May of 2005, performed by Dr. Jason Zagrodsky at Texas Cardiac Arrhythmia. I had an awesome experience (this is an incredible, cutting edge group of doctors). The procedure was successful, and I was free of A-Fib.

DEALING WITH A-FIB ANXIETY

While the heart was doing great, I dealt with a ton of anxiety which I have learned is a side effect for many heart patients.

Of the entire experience of the last ten years, anxiety has been the greatest challenge. (Don't beat yourself up if you deal with this. Be honest with the doctors about it and get help. And help your family to understand as they are your greatest support system.)

> ❖ *"Of the entire experience of the last ten years, anxiety has been the greatest challenge."*
>
> Jay Teresi

RECURRENCE OF A-FIB

All went well for three years until February of 2008 when I suddenly went into A-Fib again. (I broke my rule about stimulants and took some sinus medication. That was a mistake!)

Needless to say, I was pretty crushed. After 24 hours in the hospital, I was transported and cardioverted by the doctor who had done my original ablation. They wanted to let it go and see how things played out, which we did. For the first time I began having frequent heart palpitations which unnerved me greatly. After a month we opted for a second ablation.

SECOND ABLATION

Dr. Joseph Gallinghouse (of the same group) performed my second ablation using experimental equipment (a robotic arm, cool stuff). He explained that my first procedure was a success. However, during the healing process a tiny spot did not scar, and this allowed the A-Fib to trip again (This was the hypothesis. However, he confirmed this when he went in for the second ablation).

The procedure was a success. He ablated that portion and touched up all the other areas. My procedure and recovery were flawless, no complications whatsoever.

FREE OF A-FIB WITHOUT MEDS, BUT SOME PROBLEMS

I have now been free of A-Fib for over four years (as of September, 2011), and I am medication free. I still deal with the anxiety. And for some reason frequent heart palpitations have become part of my life. In addition, my second procedure left me with frequent heartburn (something I never had before); a side effect I have learned comes occasionally with ablation.

While I have learned that A-Fib has created some challenges for me, I have also garnered many blessings. I exercise six days a week, eat very healthy, and am in the best shape of my life at age 35. Not sure I would ever take this good care if I had not experienced A-Fib (I want to be around for my four little kids!)

> ❖ *"A-Fib is more mentally debilitating rather than physically for the young. ... The heart is a strong muscle that can often handle more than the psyche can."*
>
> Jay Teresi

LESSONS LEARNED: ADVICE FOR THE YOUNG

My advice for young A-Fib patients is if you are a candidate for ablation, go for it! Also, be gentle with yourself if you experience fear or anxiety as a result of A-Fib. (You *are* normal; you have been through a traumatic experience!)

A-Fib is more mentally debilitating rather than physically for the young. Keep that in mind! The heart is a strong muscle that can often handle more than the psyche can.

My EP here in Atlanta (Dr. Andrew Wickliffe, Piedmont Heart Institute) says it best, "Jay, you are not a guy with a heart problem. You live life and leave the A-Fib to me. It is my problem, not yours."

So try and see the blessings you have received from A-Fib and not the challenges. As a Christian I take heart in knowing that the Lord will never give me more than I can bear.

Jay Teresi
Atlanta, GA, USA

Editorial Comments:

Jay's story is somewhat unusual in that his A-Fib reoccurred after being A-Fib free for three years. Reoccurrence, if it happens, usually takes place during the first six months after an ablation.

One important lesson to be learned from Jay's story is that catheter ablations and Maze-type surgeries sometimes are not permanent. Heart tissue is very tough. There is a tendency for ablated areas to heal and reconnect. With Pulmonary Vein Isolation there is a 6%–7% chance per year of regrowth (reconnection) out to five years. Don't let this discourage you when seeking a permanent cure of your A-Fib.

Though it's unfortunate that Jay's A-Fib returned, he still had three great years of being A–Fib free. He described his second ablation as seeming simpler and easier than his first.

Anxiety and fear are unfortunate byproducts of living with Atrial Fibrillation. The threat of an A-Fib attack, the sense of fragility and powerlessness can be debilitating and unnerving, especially for younger people.

This was particularly true in Jay's case where he and his wife were raising four young children. Jay's story is important not only for his success in becoming A-Fib free, but for how he recognized but struggled with the emotional and psychological problems that often come with A-Fib.

❖

The Spouse's Perspective: A Young Wife and Mother Copes with Husband's A-Fib

Kelly married Jay Teresi just months after he had his first A-Fib attack. Today, ten years later, Kelly describes what it was like raising four children while trying to cope with her husband's Atrial Fibrillation.

A FEW MONTHS BEFORE we were married in 2001 we were entertaining friends when Jay felt his heart racing. He had had a few glasses of wine. We didn't think much of it. But when he woke up the next day, his heart was still racing. We decided to go to the ER where they figured out it was Atrial Fibrillation; they gave him some medication.

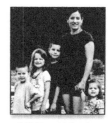

Kelly Teresi & her four kids: (L-to-R) Carter, Ayla, Aidan, Kelly and Cora. Atlanta, GA, USA

Jay became super sensitive to his heart. His A-Fib attacks triggered a kind of debilitating anxiety or panic in him.

During our honeymoon in Maui we wound up in the ER on the 4th of July. I'm not sure if it was a true episode or something triggered by a panic attack.

THE FIRST FIVE YEARS

During the first five years of our marriage we made a lot of ER visits. Medical people would tell him, "You are very young to be going through this." Hearing that didn't make me feel any better.

> ❖ *"I can't really understand the anxiety he went through all these years."*
>
> Kelly Teresi

Those early years were difficult. I was either pregnant or had a newborn. We lived near family which was helpful. It meant we could leave our kids with a family member so I could go with Jay to the ER. It was different when we moved to Georgia where we don't have family. The first few months here Jay had to go to the ER by himself because I couldn't take all the kids with me.

I can't really understand the anxiety he went through all these years. He has always provided for us, kept a very steady and successful job, and really tried hard to be all he could.

I know he had thoughts like "What if I die? What if I have a stroke or heart attack and leave my young wife and kids?"

It's still hard for me to appreciate the stress he went through.

A-FIB CASTS A LONG SHADOW OVER OUR LIVES

A-Fib was constantly in the background of our lives. Jay wouldn't go on vacation unless it was near a major hospital. If we did go somewhere, he found out exactly where the hospital was on the computer–without me knowing—just in case.

> ❖ *"A-Fib was constantly in the background of our lives."*
>
> Kelly Teresi

Over the years Jay's A-Fib became more of a

nuisance to me. It's not that I didn't believe him, because I did believe something was going on with his heart. But I didn't believe that every occurrence was an ER-related thing. There were times that his heart ended up "converting on its own" before reaching the hospital, and there was nothing the ER could do for him. At one visit the nurse told him his potassium levels were low. But each time it was another emergency doctor's bill, and those added up quickly. I got frustrated a lot, because he was so hypersensitive to ANY irregularity in his heart.

He had a blood pressure monitor, and he would check his pulse three–four times a day. He checked his blood pressure and pulse in our closet which was kind of a secret place for him to do it. I think this constant monitoring fed his anxiety. (For the last couple of months he has really worked hard on not checking it as often.)

Over the years Jay trained himself to check his pulse at his wrist for any abnormal beats. It became an automatic reflex that he did maybe five times an hour. I used to tell him, or hit him on the shoulder, "Don't do that. Stop checking your pulse." Any time his hand crossed on his lap, he would be checking his pulse on his wrist. It was just an automatic reflex that he kept doing. Now, ten years later, I will see him check his pulse but it is less than twice a day now.

> ❖ *"If there is another young wife or mother reading this, know I had a lot of resentment toward his heart issues."*
>
> Kelly Teresi

In the beginning I was trying to be very understanding. But then I was raising kids and I needed him to be a lot more mentally able to parent with me. But he was really sidetracked with his heart.

ANGER, FRUSTRATION AND RESENTMENT

If there is another young wife or mother reading this, know I had a lot of resentment toward his heart issues. I asked myself, "Why am I so frustrated?" I had a lot of anger against the way his heart condition was taking Jay away from our family. I don't like admitting that, but that was reality for me.

The biggest challenge I have had is the constant attempt to keep our family stability, even in the times I was so scared, and he was at the ER alone. I had to be the strong one that kept the kids calm and understand that we are not in control.

Our faith has been one of the biggest rocks we have ever leaned on. We continue to lean on this rock knowing that life is full of challenges; it is how you deal with the challenges that make who you are. He was constantly concerned about his heart, and that kept him from being fully present as a father and husband. I tried hard to keep the family peace and dynamics, and at different times in our parenting lives the willingness to uphold two ends of the parenting spectrum was a challenge. It took a lot of energy and patience to take on that role without really knowing I was doing it.

> ❖ *"Our faith has been one of the biggest rocks we have ever leaned on."*
>
> Kelly Teresi

At the beginning, I had no idea what living with Jay's A-Fib would be like for me. I didn't look for support either, so I can't say there wasn't any. At some point I just thought the A-Fib would stop. So I just kept going along. You kind of take it a day at a time, and just keep loving them through the challenges.

A-FIB FREE, BUT ITS IMPACT IS STILL FELT

In May 2005, after four years with A-Fib, Jay had a Pulmonary Vein Isolation procedure at the Texas Cardiac Arrhythmia Institute in Austin. As a young mom with a son and a six-weeks-old newborn daughter, I was worried. I remember I was breast feeding. The procedure was taking so long I had to leave to go pump. I was scared because doctors had told me that his heart issues increase his risk of stroke.

> ❖ *"As a young mom with a son and a six-weeks-old newborn daughter, I was worried."*
>
> Kelly Teresi

But it was successful, and Jay was A-Fib free for three years. In February 2008 though, his A-Fib returned. He had a second ablation in May 2008 and has been A-Fib free ever since.

But his A-Fib and the associated anxiety has left its imprint on our lives.

Before his A-Fib, Jay was a high energy person. But when he had A-Fib, he wouldn't exercise or lift weights. When he would wrestle with the kids on the floor, he would stop to check his pulse. I am very athletic. So I would mow the lawn and all that stuff. He would do other things which were helpful. But he didn't want to get his heart rate too high. (The doctor told him not to let his heart rate go over 180, because that would trigger his A-Fib.)

In the past year he has exerted a lot more of his energy to being physically active again, exercising, hiking, mowing the lawn, etc. (He did wear a heart rate monitor when he started the transition back to mowing the lawn.) He has made huge leaps and bounds in the last six months and isn't allowing the worry of his heart to keep him from doing things around our house.

A-FIB TRIGGERS STILL HAUNT HIM

Diet and other A-Fib triggers are still mental hurdles for Jay. He used to wear a Christian cross around his neck. But he thought the metal triggered his A-Fib. He never wore the cross again. He decided that eggs triggered his A-Fib, so he doesn't eat eggs (though he will eat something with eggs in it). Before we had kids he ate some ice cream or yogurt, then later had an A-Fib attack. He associates anything cold with A-Fib. He hasn't had a drink of alcohol in ten years, and he used to be a bartender when we were dating. The doctor told him that alcohol could trigger an A-Fib attack, so he quit that night. I think avoiding these triggers gave him some comfort over the years—that he could somewhat control his A-Fib. He is currently working very hard on overcoming the mental challenges his A-Fib has presented. I am so proud of him!

> ❖ *"Diet and other A-Fib triggers are still mental hurdles for Jay."*
>
> Kelly Teresi

A "NEW NORMAL" LIFESTYLE SLOWLY RETURNING

We were very active before getting married. We camped, etc. Then this happened. Our life took a dip. And each heart issue made the dip in our activity level a little bit lower. He gave up camping, golfing, back packing. There was a change in our personalities. We did more easy going vacations and trips. Anything with physical exertion or not near a hospital we didn't even consider doing.

Now after ten years, we are going back to where we left off. We have been camping in the mountains with no cell phone coverage, which I thought would panic him, but he did great. He even said he loved the whole trip, he enjoyed the kids, and he wasn't worried about where the hospitals were.

We've finally got a handle on his anxiety, too. Looking back I thought "Wow, it's been a while."

There was a point where I never saw a light at the end of the tunnel. But in the past year we've definitely seen the light—that our lives can get back to "a new normal"—and we are going uphill right now at a very exciting speed!

LESSONS LEARNED

I think the biggest thing I have learned, and am still learning ten years later, is to pray for patience and understanding. This disease is so far beyond what a non-A-Fib person can comprehend—many times I found myself frustrated, not understanding what was going on with Jay's thoughts and heart.

Looking back I would have urged my husband to get professional counseling. Having a heart procedure can lead to post traumatic stress and anxiety. I'm told that couple's counseling can help when one spouse feels burdened with the patience, understanding and emotional support required on behalf of the other spouse. If I had information that would have helped me to help Jay—it could have strengthened our marriage bonds and lines of communication.

Patience and love are the most important things I could think to give my husband over the years as A-Fib has been a big part of our lives. So far, in the last three–five years, we have been blessed not to have another "issue" with Jay's heart. The constant worry of A-Fib no longer affects our lives like it did, and we are very grateful for that.

Kelly Teresi
Atlanta, GA, USA

Editorial Comments:

Kelly's story reveals that anger, frustration and resentment are a normal reaction to the stress of a loved one with A-Fib.

Her first-hand account shows how Atrial Fibrillation affects more than just the patient. Family and close friends suffer the fall-out of your A-Fib; they need support and understanding as well.

Kelly mentions couples counseling to help both partners deal with issues caused by A-Fib. Sometimes it helps to share with someone else who understands what you're going through. If you'd like to correspond with an A-Fib Support Volunteer, go to A-Fib.com. Our volunteers are listed by country or region of the world. They are just an email away; they have had A-Fib and know what you're going through and offer you their support. (Note: This is a free service from A-Fib.com; volunteers receive no compensation.)

❖

A Life on Meds Wasn't Good Enough—Selects a Minimally Invasive Cox-Maze IV

Sheri didn't want a life on medication. While still in the hospital and dissatisfied with her doctor's lack of alternatives, she researched her options and found her way to a life free of both medications and her A-Fib.

IN 2006 AFTER 37 YEARS of teaching high school math in Boyce, Virginia, I retired at 59. My husband and I had just fulfilled our lifetime dream of owning a farm. We began our hay and horse boarding business, riding our horses, traveling the world and getting back into good physical shape.

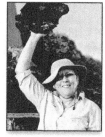

Sheri Weber
Boyce, Virginia, USA

RETIREMENT DREAM! THEN SHORTNESS OF BREATH

Then in October 2008, I had back-to-back respiratory flu which I could not seem to get over. I pushed as hard as I could but kept feeling more exhaustion, then shortness of breath, and finally a pain down my right arm that did not allow me to sleep at night. My personal trainer worried that I was moving backwards and questioned if I should even try to work out. Finally the shortness of breath was so bad I could barely walk three steps without gasping for air. I went to see my family doctor thinking I might have pneumonia. After listening to my heart and doing an EKG, the doctor ordered an immediate echo cardiogram. I was to return to his office as soon as the echo was done. He called for the results and sent me directly to the hospital indicating I had A-Fib with an extremely high risk for stroke.

> ❖ *"His response was to tell me many people live with A-Fib and did not suggest any treatment aside from medication."*
>
> Sheri Weber

JUST TAKE THE MEDS AND LIVE WITH IT

Test results showed on top of A-Fib I had a leaking mitral valve, enlarged heart, ejection fraction 30%, racing pulse and high blood pressure. The plan was to stabilize my issues with medications including Coumadin. If my heart did not convert back to NSR in a month, a cardioversion would be done.

I questioned the cardio doctor about my future with A-Fib thinking there must be a cure and knowing absolutely nothing about the disease. His response was to tell me many people live with A-Fib and did not suggest any treatment aside from medication. He talked to me about activity limitations because of the Coumadin. I faced the conclusion that my active lifestyle was completely compromised.

ELECTRICAL CARDIOVERSION

In a February '09, I returned to my cardio doctor, still in A-Fib, with all my other heart issues showing improvement.

Right before my cardioversion the PA [PHYSICIAN'S ASSISTANT] told me I needed to understand that I was in the beginning stages of congestive heart failure. I was devastated. The cardio doctor told me he guaranteed the cardioversion would put me back in NSR but made no promises about how long it would last. Now back in NSR I thought I had beaten the odds.

SOTALOL AND FLECAINIDE

I was admitted to the hospital after the electrical cardioversion for three days for the first six doses of Sotalol. The cardioversion lasted only three weeks. I was back in A-Fib and in the hospital for an increased dosage of Sotalol. My heart self-converted, but the increase in the Sotalol had unbearable side effects. I was dizzy and exhausted in addition to having issues regulating my Coumadin level. I went into A-Fib again after two weeks and ended up in the hospital again.

I refused to increase the level of Sotalol since I was feeling like an exhausted zombie. The cardio doctor switched me to flecainide. My heart self-converted, and I was thinking flecainide was a better drug choice. But flecainide worked for only a couple of weeks, and the side effects were equally as bad as Sotalol. Back in the hospital once again, I felt like I had hit rock bottom.

TREATMENT OPTIONS OTHER THAN MEDICATIONS

During this hospitalization I questioned my cardio doctor about treatment options other than medication. I also realized that I would not be able to go to on my trip to Tanzania in December. This was a trip my husband and I had planned to celebrate our 40th wedding anniversary. My cardio doctor told me there were surgical procedures, but they had very low success rates (wrong!). In addition he told me that none of the local cardio doctors would know how to take care of me if I sought a surgical solution.

> ❖ *"Anger and determination led me to spend the days in the hospital researching options on my laptop."*
>
> Sheri Weber

Anger and determination led me to spend the days in the hospital researching options on my laptop. I found two surgical options—maze and ablation. After reading about Dr. Niv Ad, a maze specialist and Dr. Sarfraz Durrani, an ablation specialist, both in Fairfax, Virginia, I made a consultation appointment with both doctors. After consulting with Dr. Duranni about an ablation, I learned that I was not a good candidate. He encouraged me to consult Dr. Niv Ad.

I found Dr. Ad to be a compassionate, soft spoken doctor who reassured me he could fix my problem with a Maze operation. In addition, Dr. Ad told me he could fix the leaking mitral valve as well.

COX-MAZE IV OPERATION

My focus was to be A-Fib free with no medication, so I asked a few questions about the surgical procedure scheduled for two weeks later. "Can you operate on me if I am in A-Fib at the time of the operation?" Dr. Ad said yes, that being in A-Fib wouldn't be a problem. "Why remove the Left Atrial Appendage (LAA)?" Dr. Ad explained that the LAA was where blood clots could form when my heart was in A-Fib, and that he would sew it shut.

The surgery revealed what seemed to be the cause of my original A-Fib.

During the procedure Dr. Ad asked his PA [PHYSICIAN'S ASSISTANT] to go and double check my records to be sure I had not had an ablation. The inside of my heart revealed scarring from a virus in my heart. This was most likely caused by the back-to-back respiratory viruses I had the previous fall. This caused Dr. Ad to adjust his original surgical plan.

The surgery lasted five hours. After two days of intensive care and two days of step down at the INOVA Fairfax Cardiovascular Institute, I walked out of the hospital to start my recovery feeling that the weight of the world had been lifted off my shoulders.

RECOVERY: A DAILY CHALLENGE

Recovery was a slow and steady process for six–eight weeks. I had to work on my breathing and try to walk as much as possible. Each day presented a new challenge, but I accepted the need to take it easy to recover. At three months, after heart Holter monitoring, I was off all medications. This was a huge step forward as I was free of Coumadin and had no more side effects from medications.

> ❖ *"I walked out of the hospital to start my recovery feeling that the weight of the world had been lifted off my shoulders."*
>
> Sheri Weber

In December my husband and I celebrated 40 years of marriage on safari in Tanzania! For the first time in a year I did not have to worry about A-Fib interfering with my plans as it had so many times in the last year.

A-FIB FREE: TWO YEARS AND COUNTING

The year I spent in A-Fib caused me to miss my niece's college graduation, my husband's retirement roast, and my daughter's visit from California. I was in A-Fib the day before the birth of my first grandchild.

Today almost two years later I am in better shape, and feel better than ever. My cardio and total body workout has surpassed where I was even before I was in A-Fib. My energy level is great. I pursue all my activities—riding horses, farm work, working out and nature adventure travel with absolutely no worries. I have hiked in high altitudes —which had been most difficult for me. Each time I work out, my cardio is better. Mentally I wake up every day able to do what I want not worrying about A-Fib or going to the hospital. I am off all drugs except Zocor for my cholesterol and Lexapro for my depression.

I am so grateful to Dr. Ad and his team at the Inova Fairfax Cardiovascular Institute for the high quality of care I received. I realize I cannot officially say I am cured forever, but I am thankful for every day I have in NSR.

LESSONS LEARNED

I wish I had realized that the *first* doctor you see is *not* necessarily the right one for you. I fooled around way too long, believing what my cardio doctor said. I should have been thinking outside the box.

Run—don't walk—to the best specialist you can find in your area. Use the internet to research A-Fib doctors and hospitals. Be aggressive. A-Fib hardly ever gets better. Find the solution that fits you best. Every case is different. You can learn from others' experiences, but you cannot determine what is best for your case unless you have all the facts, tests and personal goals in line.

> ❖ *"Run–don't walk–to the best specialist you can find in your area."*
>
> Sheri Weber

My health has been great. But now that I have

solved the big issue, I realize I need to keep up on the other appropriate health tests for my age. During my year of A-Fib, I could only focus on that. Now it is time to move on and be aggressive about protecting my complete health.

Sheri Weber
Boyce, Virginia, USA

Editorial Comments:
Sheri Weber had a "Minimally Invasive Cox-Maze IV" operation using Cryo (freezing) lesions (rather than RF lesions). Though she was on heart-lung bypass, it was not an open chest operation. Instead of cracking open the breastbone, small keyhole incisions were made between the ribs to access her heart and perform the surgery with video-guided instruments.

Unlike Sheri's first cardiologist, most cardiologists today will refer their A-Fib patients to an electrophysiologists (EP) to discuss a catheter ablation procedure, and then perhaps to a cardiac surgeon to consider a surgical treatment option.

Today's catheter ablations and surgical options offer the best hope of a permanent cure for A-Fib. But to get there sometimes you need to be angry enough to do your own research, like Sheri did, to find your cure.

In 2000 Chooses a Full Surgical Cox-Maze (Open Chest), Three Generations with A-Fib

Roger, a former U.S. Marine, watched his father cope with Atrial Fibrillation and then developed it himself. In 2000, at age 65, he had a full (open chest) surgical Cox-Maze. In hindsight, he thinks he may have rushed into that decision to avoid going on Coumadin. Since then, cardio health challenges continued to unfold for him, including his daughter developing A-Fib.

I INHERITED ATRIAL FIBRILLATION from my father. I watched my father cope with irregular heartbeat for which he took Digoxin and had several cardioversions. So when I started to notice my own irregular heartbeat in my late 30s or early 40s, I had some understanding of it. Seeking treatment at that time, I was informed that A-Fib was basically a nuisance and that it would not kill me. I was informed that many lived long successful lives with it including a local former senator who was nearing 90 years of age. I began a regimen of Digoxin.

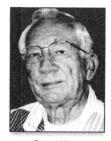

Roger Meyer
Columbus, Ohio, USA

I tended to be a pretty active person and loved tennis and especially the game of four-wall handball, playing four or five times a week for decades. The cardiologist kept advising me along the way that at some point I would have to start Coumadin. But I understood that with Coumadin I would no longer be able to play handball due to the bruising of the hands that would result. I continually protested that I was too active and was caring for myself with exercise. I felt I could put off Coumadin. By age 60 I had also taken up crew/rowing and loved it.

> ❖ *"Episodes...became a part of my life—just as I had watched my dad cope with his A-Fib."*
>
> Roger Meyer

As the years passed my heart irregularity did not. I remember times at the gym where I would have to lay on the bench in front of my locker to let the A-Fib episode pass. I used to love drinking Pepsi—many times poured from a two liter bottle. That began to be a trigger for A-Fib, and so I had to change my taste in soft drinks to less caffeine. Episodes of irregularity came and went, and it just became a part of my life—just as I had watched my dad cope with his A-Fib.

Gradually, my Digoxin dosage was increased to the point that I was on .375 mg which I came to understand is a rather high dosage level. But for me it took that much dosage with my basal metabolism to have sufficient residual level to keep my heart irregularity reasonably under control. With regular check-ups by my cardiologist (plumber type), my seeming good overall health continued satisfactorily.

> ❖ *"But as I approached 60 years of age, I started to notice how I would break into a sweat very easily."*
>
> Roger Meyer

But as I approached 60 years of age, I started to notice how I would break into a sweat very easily. I remember when I had to walk to professional meetings in another building on campus, I would have to start walking there early so I could walk slowly enough as to not be sweat-wet in my dress clothes as I arrived for the meeting. That was becoming a problem for me. I forget now when Cardizem was added to my regimen. My dosage was 180mg.

COUMADIN OR THE COX-MAZE?

In 2000, as I reached the age of 65, my cardiologist became insistent and gave me an ultimatum that I had to start Coumadin. My cardiologist was a good guy who had played handball himself, so he understood my reluctance. He also told me there was a surgical option I could consider instead of starting Coumadin. It was the Cox-Maze procedure [THE ORIGINAL OPEN-CHEST FULL COX-MAZE SURGERY] that Dr. Cox had just brought to Ohio State University [WHERE ROGER ALSO WORKED]. He had performed ten Maze procedures working with local cardio thoracic surgeons.

> ❖ *"I expected to be in and out of the hospital in a week or ten days —but that was not to be the case."*
>
> Roger Meyer

I think I may have somewhat rushed into the notion of the surgery in order to avoid Coumadin. I had the surgery scheduled during the month of August [2000]. I expected to be in and out of the hospital in a week or ten days and would be ready for Ohio State's football season—but that was not to be the case.

COX-MAZE SURGERY WITH UNEXPECTED TURN

The operation itself went quite well. I recovered quickly and was able to walk the cardio floor loop up to fourteen times in one day (while pulling along my IV pole). I was very pleased with my recovery; although I recall that the EP would come into my room periodically, check the monitor and observe that no "P waves" were yet noted. That seemed to be discouraging to him and to my case for NSR.

But my good early recovery took an unwelcome turn, and it took some time for them to figure out what was happening. It turned out that instead of my being hospitalized for seven to ten days, I was there in excess of three weeks.

SECOND SURGERY RE-OPENS CHEST

It was finally determined that I had a pericardial effusion (a sac of blood pressing on the heart). An attempt was made in the EP lab to deal with this, but it was unsuccessful. Then I was wheeled directly into urgent surgery and my chest re-opened to deal with the effusion.

> ❖ *"Then I was wheeled directly into urgent surgery and my chest re-opened to deal with the effusion."*
>
> Roger Meyer

RECOVERY SLOWED BY SEPSIS INFECTION

My recovery was slower this time. In the course of recovery I eventually developed sepsis (staphylococcus infection throughout my body's system). I was in a very weakened state after having started with a strong recovery from the Maze. I was discharged, but for six weeks I had to perform self-infusions of antibiotics at home to treat the sepsis.

Recovery continued slowly, but I got my strength back, gradually walking more paces daily—always mindful that energy for the distance walked had to allow for equal energy for the distance required to walk back.

END RESULT OF COX-MAZE—NOT IN NSR

The end result of my Maze was that I did NOT return to NSR [NORMAL SINUS RHYTHM]. Instead I was determined to be operating in "junctional rhythm" where the pacing is done from the node at the junction between the atrial and ventricle chambers. While not in NSR, I returned to my previous lifestyle. I was able to walk to the top deck of the football stadium for the football games, return to the gym and resume crew/rowing. Life was good!

> ❖ *"The end result of my Maze was that I did NOT return to NSR (normal sinus rhythm)."*
>
> Roger Meyer

HOLTER MONITORING LEADS TO PACEMAKER

The following June [2001], my heart decided to "talk" to me with strange strong/pounding beats that were very different from anything I had had previously! My cardiologist had me wear the Holter Monitor. After I turned it in, his office worked frantically to get in contact with me to tell me I needed to come to the hospital *immediately* for a pacemaker implant. My heart rate was ranging, without my sensing it, from very high rates to very slow rates with up to eight seconds between beats.

Thus, I received my first pacemaker. I recall while I was under the "sanitary tent" while the EP was implanting the pacer, he admonished me for not yet being on Coumadin. I recall arguing with him that Coumadin was not needed because with my Maze, the Left Atrial Appendage (LAA) had been removed. I recall he was not impressed, but I let him win that one at the time.

TIA EVEN WITH LAA REMOVED

It turned out that he was right. In time I experienced a Transient Ischemic Attack (TIA). The symptoms of a TIA are the same as a stroke, in my case, speech interruption (aphasia). But unlike a stroke which is permanent, a TIA resolves on its own. After that I was advised by my regular cardiologist (plumber type) to start Coumadin which I finally did.

SICK SINUS SYNDROME & NON-FUNCTIONING ATRIUM

Due to the many years in A-Fib before my Maze procedure, my diagnosis included "sick sinus syndrome." The diagnosis of SSS was "after the fact" and after I had my pacer implanted. It is why I was given a single chamber pacer with a lead only to the ventricle and no lead to the atrium.

I could not sense my "nonfunctioning atrium." It was basically sitting there and "quivering" and not being productive. So, I can now say, first hand, that there ARE bad effects from A-Fib and especially from A-Fib that is not treated early. I now wish I had had some of the today's more aggressive A-Fib treatment options which weren't available to me in my younger years.

> ❖ *"...there ARE bad effects from A-Fib and especially from A-Fib that is not treated early."*
>
> Roger Meyer

MY PACEMAKER BUDDY

My pacemaker batteries only lasted seven years (the average is ten years). At which point I received my current pacer, still a single chamber pacer (because of my sick sinus syndrome). I like to call my pacer my "buddy"—I can basically do what I want—my lifestyle continues to include racquetball, although my knees are now "talking" to me and reminding me of my years.

AV NODE ABLATION AND PACER DEPENDENT

During 2010, I complained to my cardiologist of another heart health development—"racing heartbeat runs" that would come and go. I would notice them when I was sitting in office meetings, or when I was at my desk, or watching TV, etc. and wonder what was going on again! After evaluation and consulting with EPs, an AV Node Ablation was done in January, 2011. That took care of these racing heartbeat episodes, and I am now considered "pacer dependent." I learned, however, that if my pacemaker fails, my heart still has rudimentary pacing that will support me getting to the hospital for treatment.

IS CONGESTIVE HEART FAILURE NEXT?

After the AV Node Ablation, my recent Echocardiogram revealed that my ejection fraction had reduced to 35% from the consistently previous 55%–65%. [EJECTION FRACTION, I.E., THE ABILITY OF THE HEART TO PUMP, IS NORMALLY 55%–70%] I have learned that can happen from a single chamber pacer that over time can change the pumping profile of the ventricle chamber.

I have also learned that the next likely step of my cardio health is the probable development of "congestive heart failure." Sad and bad as that term sounds, I have learned it is a treatable "syndrome" and does not mean a relatively fast end of life as the term can imply. It is a cardio condition that can logically evolve in a case like mine.

> ❖ "...the probable development of "congestive heart failure." Sad and bad as that term sounds, I have learned it is a treatable 'syndrome'."
>
> Roger Meyer

I also learned that further possible treatment is the implanting of a new pacer that will also have a defibrillator capability. At this point I don't know what the scheduling of these possibilities is. My next echocardiogram will tell me more.

MY ATTITUDE AND QUALITY OF LIFE

As to my overall quality of life, past and present, you may have to ask those around me. They see me as a Type-A person. I am active. One would not know I had cardio challenges including a pacemaker unless they were informed.

I do wear a Medic-Alert bracelet. But when I am at the gym, I put my wrist sweat band over it so my partners don't have to be concerned about me as a cardio guy. They do not know I have a pacemaker, and I don't really want them to know. I don't want them to cut me any slack either! Racquetball anyone?

LESSONS LEARNED

I am the oldest of three sons, and as it turns out all of us have A-Fib. I keep my brothers informed of my ongoing status and they about theirs.

My youngest of two daughters is also diagnosed with A-Fib. Starting with my dad, that makes three generations of my family with A-Fib. My daughter is currently 38 years of age and has two young children, and I am left to wonder as the years pass whether A-Fib will evidence itself in that generation as well. I hope not.

I encourage our daughter to stay in close contact with her cardiologist so she can avoid what I have experienced. There are so many treatments available today for early intervention, and I applaud that. I urge my daughter and others to seek treatment early and follow through with whatever is wisely advised.

> ❖ *"I urge my daughter and others [with A-Fib] to seek treatment early and follow through with whatever is wisely advised."*
>
> Roger Meyer

In retrospect, even though I still ended up on Coumadin, I am glad I had the Cox- Maze surgery. I now regard the various "next steps" of my cardio challenges as the normal progression of my heart disease. My great cardio team kept me informed of my choices and offered their recommendations along the way to help me make my decisions.

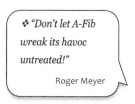

> ❖ *"Don't let A-Fib wreak its havoc untreated!"*
>
> Roger Meyer

I still feel the Cox-Maze was an appropriate choice for me at the time I had to make my decision. My Maze was done at The Ohio State University Medical Center, and now the Center has the new Ross Heart Hospital with a phenomenal number of cardiologists and cardio thoracic procedures from which to choose. I wish that array of options was available to me when I needed to make my choice.

My best advice: Don't let A-Fib wreak its havoc untreated!

Roger Meyer
Columbus, Ohio, USA

Editorial Comments:

Most Cox-Maze surgeries, though traumatic and invasive, usually produce better results than in Roger's case. Not only was he not in Normal Sinus Rhythm (NSR) after the surgery, but somehow in the surgery the Sinus Node/AV Node Junction was compromised (no P waves). Then he had to have a second open heart surgery to take care of a pericardial effusion, and he developed Sepsis which is an infection that can kill you.

Even though he had his Left Atrial Appendage (LAA) closed off, he still had a TIA (Mini-Stroke) — this is unusual and troubling. Effectively removing the LAA normally reduces the danger of stroke when in A-Fib.

Needing a pacemaker does occasionally happen after a Cox-Maze type surgery. But having an AV Node Ablation to stop racing heartbeats is usually a strategy of last resort.

It's not surprising that Roger is faced with the threat of Congestive Heart Failure (CHF). But what is surprising is Roger's attitude—he is an inspiration for anyone with more complex heart problems.

❖

A-Fib Burden Lifted After Consulting a New Cardiologist Down Under

Aussie Warren's first cardiologist was critical of catheter ablation. When the burden of his A-Fib worsened, he did his own online research and decided to change cardiologists. He got the ablations he needed, and now for the first time since 1998 he's A-Fib free.

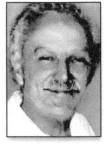

Warren Welsh
Melbourne, Australia

MY NAME IS WARREN Welsh from Melbourne, Australia. I was diagnosed with paroxysmal A-Fib back in 1998, at the age of 60, when I consulted my doctor after detecting an irregular pulse during a heavy bout of influenza. I was then referred to a cardiologist who confirmed I had PAF (paroxysmal A-Fib) and prescribed a low dose of Sotalol.

Though I had regained normal sinus rhythm within 24 hours, he advised it was more than likely the episodes would become longer and more frequent as the condition itself worsens with age, eventually progressing to a chronic state. By 2003, 40–50 hour periods of A-Fib were occurring three or four times a year and after 2005 the occurrences had almost doubled.

After purchasing a computer in 2005, I became a regular visitor to A-Fib.com. The personal experiences and the successful outcome of the treatments available caused me to decide on an ablation. I went back to my cardiologist in late 2006 to discuss the prospect of an ablation. To my surprise he spoke critically of the procedure and advised against it.

THE BURDEN WORSENS, CHANGES DOCTORS

By 2009 the A-Fib had become such a burden that I decided to consult a different cardiologist and was referred to Dr. Joe Morton, an electrophysiologist who booked me into Royal Melbourne Hospital for an ablation in March 2010. All went smoothly under general anesthesia, apart from a short bout of A-Fib in the recovery room; I was in NSR (Normal Sinus Rhythm) on discharge.

> ❖ *"By 2009 the A-Fib had become such a burden that I decided to consult a different cardiologist."*
>
> Warren Welsh

One month post ablation I had a bout of A-Fib which lasted only 15 hours followed by a much shorter episode of just eight hours two months later. Despite the substantial improvement achieved by Dr. Joe Morton, a "new" more gentle type of A-Fib had emerged eight months after the procedure occurring several times a day. Curiously, on most occasions, I was able to terminate the bouts with moderate exercise. Nonetheless it became clear I would need to arrange a second ablation as soon as possible.

SUBSTANTIAL IMPROVEMENT BUT REQUIRES SECOND ABLATION

Unfortunately the waiting list at Royal Melbourne Hospital had extended well beyond six months, and I was not prepared to wait that long. Late in 2010, I wrote to Steve Ryan explaining my situation and asking for advice on which electrophysiologists I might approach. As luck would have it, one of the first on the list he provided, Dr. Rukshen Weerasooriya, had an ablation vacancy at the Royal Perth Hospital on the 27th January, 2011, which I immediately accepted.

I was sedated in the O.R. and conscious during the procedure and aware of what was happening. Within a short period of time the problem area was located and ablated. Before discharge the following morning Dr. Weerasooriya attended me and advised that the heart monitor had not detected any arrhythmia overnight. He prescribed a daily dose of Sotalol, (divided 80 mg) and one Cartia tablet (aspirin), to be taken until such time as I could be assessed three months later; I was then cleared to fly home to Melbourne.

The only discomfort I experienced after both procedures was laying on my back on the hospital beds overnight, a measure employed to limit movement and help prevent bleeding from the incision made in the groin for the catheter entry. As expected there was some light chest pain during the first 48 hours after the procedures.

MY NEW LIFE, A-FIB FREE!

There have been so many improvements to my life since the ablation. I hardly know where to start. After 13 years of beta blocker medication, I am free from the side effects. I no longer have to avoid the many triggers peculiar to my A-Fib. I no longer worry that my next episode will be the one that would not return me to NSR. There's a dramatic increase in my exercise tolerance, and nights of uninterrupted sleep have returned as well.

> ❖ *"I no longer worry that my next episode will be the one that would not return me to NSR."*
>
> Warren Welsh

All these things have contributed to an improved quality of life. Not to mention my feelings of good fortune and gratitude for having been treated successfully. I feel great.

It is seven months since my second procedure, and I have remained free of A-Fib. It still seems like a miracle that not only was my arrhythmia arrested, but also the associated problem of a slow basal heart rate (below 40 bpm) was returned to normal. My gratitude goes to Doctors Joe Morton and Rukshen Weerasooriya for their expertise in performing the ablations.

I congratulate Steve Ryan on his exhaustive work in the creation of his most informative website (www.A-Fib.com) and thank fellow A-Fib sufferers who contributed their A-Fib personal experiences.

LESSONS LEARNED

I would urge any A-Fib sufferers not to make the same mistakes I did by not researching their treatment options. I am sure had I owned a computer when first diagnosed with A-Fib, I would have trawled the internet immediately; I would have sought an ablation much sooner.

In the early years of my A-Fib, I had made enquiries into the possibility of catheter treatment after hearing that certain types of heart flutter were being treated successfully. However, in Australia the acceptance of catheter ablation to cure A-Fib and the necessary experience and expertise in treating A-Fib lagged behind both the USA and France.

> ❖ *"I believe...any advice*
> *on treatment that is not*
> *directed towards a*
> *possible cure should be*
> *questioned."*
>
> Warren Welsh

After getting online in 2006, I was drawn to the A-Fib.com website where the author, Steve Ryan, had written of his own successful treatment in Bordeaux, France in 1998. Then later, after the FDA had sanctioned the procedure, I was convinced that it was time for me to pursue the treatment, and now I'm A-Fib free.

I experienced several years of unnecessary suffering by accepting an opinion of one specialist who said I would have to live in A-Fib. I believe that unless there are special circumstances that might preclude ablation, any advice on treatment that is not directed towards a possible cure should be questioned.

Warren Welsh
Melbourne, Australia

Editorial Comments:

We don't know why Warren's first ablation wasn't completely successful. (It should be noted that Dr. Weerasooriya received his training and worked at the French Bordeaux group which is considered by many as the best in the world.) Warren notes that his life did improve after his first ablation; this gave him the fortitude to go for his second, successful ablation.

Warren's story demonstrates how an informed patient, one who is an active participant in his own treatment, makes a world of difference. In this case—leading to a life free of A-Fib.

After eight years on meds, Warren's A-Fib burden worsened with no relief in sight from his cardiologist. Aided by his growing knowledge of A-Fib and bolstered by networking online with other A-Fib patients, he took control and made some changes. What was his first step? Change cardiologists! His actions led to choices beyond a life saddled with A-Fib, choices beyond ineffective medications. His actions lead to a life free of the burden and stress of A-Fib.

❖

First in Denial, then Pill-in-the-Pocket Served Her Well for Years

Joan's A-Fib crept slowly into her life, her second episode not occurring until four years after the first. But each year that followed had an increasing number of episodes until a new cardiologist recommended a treatment change. Today she is free of A-Fib.

MOST OF US never forget our first major A-Fib episode, and I'm no exception. My life changed that night awakened by the erratic and violent pounding in my chest. Panic began to set in accompanied by shortness of breath and pain radiating up my neck. The anxiety was overwhelming. What was happening to me?

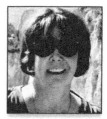

Joan Schneider
Ann Arbor, MI, USA

2001: MY FIRST ATTACK

With an erratic heart rate over 170 bpm, I made my way to the local community ER. I was experiencing Atrial Fibrillation. Tests revealed that my Potassium was low, and presumed to be the cause of my A-Fib. I was given Potassium and Diltiazem IV, and I converted to NSR in seven hours. I left the ER with a prescription for Coumadin, Cardizem and an appointment at a local larger hospital for a Stress Echo. Everything checked out great...no other apparent heart complications.

On my first appointment with the cardiologist he explained what A-Fib was, how it affected the heart, and that I would not drop dead of this to my great relief. His recommendation at the time was to keep me on Coumadin and Cardizem in the event of another episode. However, he was not impressed to find out that I did not fill the prescriptions, and I refused to start the meds. I'm not going to lie....I was in denial. I chalked this episode up to "low Potassium." I'm 41 years old! I'm not eating rat poison!

2005: SECOND EPISODE

Four years later here we go again! Second episode. The beginning of the beast. It hit in the evening and lasted two hours. Saw my GP the next day. She prescribed Atenolol 50 mg daily for rate control, and daily aspirin. Six months later, episode three, 90 minutes long. One month later, episode four, 60 minutes long. Atenolol seemed to help some with the duration of episodes.

2006: PAROXYSMAL A-FIB SETS IN

The first six episodes of this year all lasted between 50–90 minutes. I still took Atenolol 50 mg per day along with Potassium and Magnesium supplements with onset. "If these episodes last an average of an hour, I think I can live with this." But oh no...the next episode was two hours, the next three hours, and finally the last episode I had to go to the ER to be converted via Diltiazem. The ER physician explained I was now a paroxysmal A-Fibber and

> ❖ *"The ER physician explained I was now a paroxysmal A-Fibber and should consider other long term medications."*
>
> Joan Schneider

should consider other long term medications.

2007: PILL-IN-THE-POCKET (PIP)

First episode of the year (one month since last episode), I had to return to the ER after five hours to be converted once again via Diltiazem. I was then scheduled to consult with an EP.

I could no longer be in denial of this beast. My quality of life was being compromised. Two more episodes occurred prior to my appointment with the EP, all lasting up to five hours. I could not get that appointment fast enough! There had to be something they could do for me.

The EP could not believe I was aware of when I went in and out of A-Fib, and asked how I knew I was having an episode. I described my symptoms, the violent pounding, shortness of breath, pain up my sternum to my throat, horrible anxiety, and urgency to urinate every 10–15 minutes (he had no idea what this meant). I questioned him what options I had and where this was going...to my dismay, he had no real answers. He felt I was not a candidate for Ablation, and the medications he could offer would require hospitalization and were not good long term for someone my age. The only good news he had was that I did not need to be on Coumadin, and that Aspirin would be fine. We scheduled another appointment for six months down the road, and I left discouraged.

> ❖ *"I questioned him what options I had and where this was going...to my dismay, he had no real answers."*
>
> Joan Schneider

While waiting to check out, my EP tapped me on the shoulder. He handed me two new prescriptions, stating that maybe we could try this. The first was for Cardizem 240 mg/day (rate control), the second was for Rythmol 450 mg (antiarrhythmic) to be taken at the onset of an episode (the Pill-in-the-Pocket treatment). And I was to stop the Atenolol. "OK. Feeling a little better now. Don't feel appointment was a total waste."

Fourth episode of year wasn't too bad, only two hours, and much milder. No urgency to urinate, or climb the walls. This Pill-in-the-Pocket may be helping. Next episode 1.5 hours, and the last two fairly mild. And that's two less episodes than last year.

2008: P-I-P SEEMS TO BE WORKING

Continued with Cardizem for rate control and Rythmol for Pill-in-the-Pocket at onset. No episode over two hours in length and fairly mild. Seems to be working well. Wish I had seen the EP earlier.

2009: TIME TO CONSIDER OTHER TREATMENT OPTIONS

My current EP dropped me due to my insurance carrier. I am now seeing a new EP at a larger university. This is OK, another opinion is always good. I met with my new EP after having three episodes so far this year. His recommendation was to drop the Pill-in-the-Pocket, and to start Rythmol SR 325 mg 2xday and to continue with the 240 mg of Cardizem.

The next twelve episodes (over a six month period) increased in length from one hour to 14 hours! STOPPED Rythmol SR! Went back to Pill-in-the-Pocket (PIP)! The following 14 episodes decreased from 13 hours in duration, back to 1.5 hours.

It would appear this method works best for me in limiting the duration of the episodes; however, they are occurring more often. Herein lies the true nature of the Beast.

❖ *"...the episodes....are occurring more often. Herein lies the true nature of the Beast."*

Joan Schneider

Time to look into other options once again. My new EP has suggested I have an ablation, and that I am a great candidate (make up your minds!). Upon questioning him regarding the procedure, I didn't have a warm fuzzy feeling. However, I found everything I needed to know (and even what I didn't want to know) when I came across A-Fib.com, Stopafib.org, and the best support from the A-Fib support group. [SEE APPENDIX B FOR ONLINE SUPPORT GROUPS]. It was a true experience of input, input, input!

❖ *"After educating myself...my choices came down to three.... . My first step was to interview each facility by phone."*

Joan Schneider

After educating myself on all types of A-Fib, medication and surgical options, I found I needed an opinion outside of my area. My choices came down to three—Cleveland Clinic, Ohio State and Northwestern Memorial. Oddly enough, all three are about a four hour drive from home. My first step was to interview each facility by phone. I was impressed with the responses I had received from all three. However, once again I had an insurance issue, and having medical treatment out of state would be difficult. So everything was on hold for now.

2010: THE BEAST IS PROGRESSING

Despite suffering 52 episodes this year, it was a real eye opener to this disease. This disease's ultimate goal is to become chronic/permanent. I didn't want to go there. Pill-in-the-Pocket kept the episodes to less than four hours; however, they were becoming too frequent—sometimes twice in a day. I once tried no Rythmol at the onset and suffered a nine-hour episode. The Pill-in-the-Pocket did make a difference. I was now waiting for the first of the year when my new insurance will allow me to shop for a cure free of medications.

❖ *"I was short of breath, felt like my legs weighed 100 lb. a piece, and generally felt awful on Multaq."*

Joan Schneider

2011: A NEW BEGINNING

I had 13 episodes in January alone.... wow! My EP decided to place me on Multaq 400 mg (another antiarrhythmic) twice a day, along with the 240 mg of Cardizem to try and slow the episodes down. Unfortunately it did nothing; 15 episodes in February and getting longer in duration. Not to mention I was short of breath, felt like my legs weighed 100 lb. a piece, and generally felt awful on Multaq. I was definitely motivated to get this fixed.

The first two centers I contacted were the Cleveland Clinic and Ohio State. Both appeared to be good choices. However upon a week's vacation in Chicago, I called to see if the team at Northwestern Memorial Hospital (NMH) could possibly squeeze me in for a consultation. I had spoken with Jane Kruse (Nurse Coordinator) the year before and was very impressed with the time and patience she spent with me on the phone. And now she was again just as accommodating.

I met with the team at NMH on February 16th, consisting of Jane Kruse, Dr. Richard Lee (cardiac surgeon), and Dr. Rod Passman (EP). I can not express the breath of fresh air this group was. They spent over an hour of their time explaining and covering all options, and what options they felt would work for me. Then I heard the magic words "we will fix you...you will be off all meds." OK, I'm up for the challenge. I had a warm fuzzy feeling!

The choice of procedures was an ablation. Dr. Passman would perform it. The first thing he did at the consultation was to take me off of the Multaq, and place me immediately on Pradaxa (blood thinner) 150 mg 2xday because of my almost daily A-Fib episodes now. The ablation was scheduled for March 8th. It couldn't come quick enough, even though it was only three weeks away. I was ready.

ABLATION FOR MY A-FIB AND FLUTTER

My ablation took just over eight hours long. While ablating for A-Fib, a little Flutter joined in. Dr. Passman was able to take care of both, hence the length in time. He felt very positive that the procedure would leave good results. From my perspective, I felt like nothing happened at all. I was not sore really—mild groin discomfort, no chest pain, nothing. I felt pretty darn good! I drove the five-hour trip home next morning with no problems.

> ❖ *"I drove the 5-hour trip home next morning with no problems."*
>
> Joan Schneider

Once home and settled, I had an hour of A-Fib. "Oh no!" The next day I was in and out of A-Fib all day. This went on for the next two and half weeks—complete disappointment. Episodes were more frequent and severe than prior to the procedure. I tried to remain optimistic. Give myself time to heal. (*I'm told episodes are common during the three month recovery period following a PVI.*)

On March 26th I experienced a violent episode of A-Fib. I was gravely disappointed and almost went to the ER. But, I have not had any symptoms since—it went out with a bang!

QUALITY OF LIFE RESTORED

It has been six months since my last episode, and I'm currently drug free! My quality of life has been restored after ten long years! PIP served me well prior to my procedure, and I hope to buy some good time from it. I know A-Fib might rear its ugly head again. However, I feel I have chosen a great team to work with, if or when it occurs again.

LESSONS LEARNED

After very symptomatic A-Fib episodes, my quality of life has drastically changed for the better. I lived and put up with this for so long prior to my procedure, I had not realized just how much it had stolen from me.

Everything revolved around an episode. "When was one due? Has it been a day since the last episode? Do I have any drugs in my pocket? Schedule that appt earlier in the day... most episodes occur later in the day!"

> ❖ *"I had not realized just how much it [A-Fib] had stolen from me."*
> Joan Schneider

Just a few things I can now do without going into an episode: Hysterically laugh, sneeze, sleep on any side or position besides my right side, work a 16 hour day, watch a movie at a theater with loud bass, ride a roller coaster, exercise, wear out my 20-year-old children hiking in the Grand Canyon, go 0 - 80 mph in four sec in my Corvette. Not to mention the 15 lbs lost due to discontinuing the drugs (CVS Pharmacy misses me, too!). I have three times the energy that has been missing for the last five years! I can not express how great it is to have my life back!

My advice to other AF patients: Know that paroxysmal AF becomes chronic. Drugs only work for so long. Heart modification will occur, and options will become few. Get with a great EP /AF clinic and find your cure.

Personally, I will do anything to not be on drugs. I don't respond well to drugs. If there is a side effect, I will have it. If there isn't one, I will trend set one! I'm not sure which is worse, an episode or the effects of drugs I'm using to try and stop an episode.

> ❖ *"I'm not going to lie... I had a full blown panic attack the morning of my procedure."*
> Joan Schneider

Ultimately I chose an ablation. This was not chosen lightly, and I took three years to do so. I'm not going to lie... I had a full blown panic attack the morning of my procedure. But I had faith in my journey here, and ultimately made the right choice.

I wish I had found A-Fib.com, Stopafib.org and AFIBsupport groups on-line a lot sooner.

I suffered my first five years not understanding anything. I went through two cardiologists, and three EPs without ever understanding A-Fib. Just blank stares and a pat on the back. I was so desperate for answers I started searching on-line. My jaw hit the table. "How could my physicians not explain these things to me?" Once I was able to really comprehend my future, I was able to make things happen.

Best advice: Don't be afraid to fire your physician, and be your own advocate.

Joan Schneider
Ann Arbor, Michigan, USA

Editorial Comments:

Joan's story illustrates how helpful the Pill-in-the-Pocket strategy can be. Unfortunately it's often only a stop gap—a temporary measure—rather than a "cure." For many, the Pill-in-the-Pocket strategy may only postpone the inevitable choice of ablation or surgery. Remember, over time, A-Fib can remodel the heart making it more difficult to treat or cure. For this reason, most electrophysiologists today recommend that patients aim to be A-Fib free as reasonably soon as possible.

Joan's ablation took eight hours, a long time for a typical catheter ablation. After ten years in A-Fib, Joan's heart probably had many different sources of A-Fib signals. It takes time to track them all down and ablate/isolate them. We can only wonder if use of the Pill-in-the-Pocket strategy may have led to or contributed to A-Fib remodeling in her heart.

Her advice to others with A-Fib practically screams out at you—educate yourself about A-Fib— don't be afraid to fire your doctor and get another—be your own best patient advocate. She delayed doing this and suffered five additional years before seeking her A-Fib cure. Once she understood her disease, she made things happen. Today she's A-Fib free and delighted with her returned qualify of life.

Heart Attacks & Bypass Surgeries But A-Fib free After CryoBalloon Ablation

Ken developed A-Fib in 1992 post-op in the Intensive Care Unit (ICU) following quad bypass heart surgery. Controlled with medication for 15 years, a second bypass surgery ignited his A-Fib once again. Finally, in 2010, he found his cure through a CryoBalloon ablation procedure.

LIKE ALL PEOPLE who have experienced A-Fib I have found it the most frustrating, distressing and debilitating problem. Now, after having had my first A-Fib episode in 1992, I am A-Fib free. I would like to share my experience with other sufferers. If nothing else, it might provide some hope and at least give some strength to face what is an absolutely lousy problem that is almost swept under the carpet.

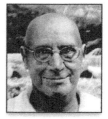

Ken Hungerford
New South Wales, Australia

IN THE BEGINNING: THE FIRST 15 YEARS

I remember my first episode as if it were yesterday. I had just returned to the medical ward after having spent two days in ICU following quad bypass heart surgery in late 1992 and was feeling surprisingly well. Suddenly my heart seemed to go crazy—rapid changes in pulse rate, palpitations and soreness in the chest. My first thought was that I was having another heart attack. Nurses quickly diagnosed it as A-Fib and brought it under control. I was placed on a drug called Rhythmodan, and all seemed to settle down.

> ❖ *"During this period I asked three cardiologists about these episodes, and they all basically told me to simply put up with them."*
>
> Ken Hungerford

For the next 15 years I only had rare episodes, usually late at night or early in the morning. They probably occurred about every two months and would only last 30 to 40 minutes.

During this period I asked three cardiologists about these episodes, and they all basically told me to simply put up with them. Even in 2010, I had doctors tell me not to worry—A-Fib does not kill you. *Of course, this is both right and wrong.* The A-Fib doesn't kill you but the resultant stroke might!

SECOND CORONARY SURGERY

During the first few months of 2008, the episodes became more severe and more frequent, but still lasted less than an hour. Then, in April 2008 I suffered another heart attack necessitating my second round of bypass surgery to redo the graft done first time around. I did know that the grafts would not last for ever; but when I was told I would have to have CABG surgery [CORONARY ARTERY BYPASS GRAFT] again, I was devastated.

I found the first surgery to be far less traumatic than I thought it would be, but the second left me very distressed and depressed. I had been warned about the additional risk but was not prepared for four days in ICU, a second visit to the operating room theatre because of bleeding, and then kidneys and liver that didn't want to recover; then—a worry that I had suffered from a minor stroke. I really don't want to go through that again.

Anyway, I survived.

DIAGNOSED WITH BOTH ATRIAL FLUTTER AND A-FIB

And around six weeks after discharge from the hospital, I started rehab classes. I had only been going several days when one morning while using the treadmill, my heart rate suddenly went to almost 140 bpm, and even after ten minutes of rest remained at over 120.

I was "escorted" to the ER and quickly diagnosed with both Atrial Flutter and A-Fib.

Regular doses of amiodarone brought the arrhythmias under control, and I was told to see my cardiologist ASAP. Around September 2008 after seeing my cardiologist, my medication was changed from amiodarone to Sotalol together with Aspirin. He explained that amiodarone was a very toxic drug, and no patient should remain on it for very long.

> ❖ *"He explained that amiodarone was a very toxic drug, and no patient should remain on it for very long."*
>
> Ken Hungerford

For the next 10–12 months I continued to have mild episodes of A-Fib. Then just prior to my cardiologist visit in September 2009, they became worse. After wearing a Holter monitor for five days which clearly showed both the Flutter and A-Fib, and being placed on warfarin, it was suggested that I make an appointment with an EP to talk about ablation. The EP seemed loathe to do anything about it at the time but did explain the ablation options. Given later actions, I still do not understand why he didn't take any action then.

> ❖ *"...the episodes became far more frequent...they were now occurring every second day."*
>
> Ken Hungerford

ABLATION BUT FOR FLUTTER

During the first few months of 2010 the episodes became far more frequent, distressing and debilitating. Whereas previously they occurred once every couple of months, lasted perhaps 45 minutes and were not too severe, they were now occurring every second day, lasting up to several hours and were very distressing in their severity. In May 2010 after being fed up with being listless, having a light head, headaches and being totally wiped out, I called my cardio and made an appointment.

As soon as he heard what I had to say, he called the EP and asked him to carry out an ablation as soon as he could. Initially I assumed that he would be able to tackle both the flutter and A-Fib at the same time.

Unfortunately, he decided to only do the Flutter.

On 22nd July I entered the hospital around 7:30 AM, was out to it by 1 PM and back in the ward by 3 PM. When I came to, I immediately felt that things had improved. The procedure used RF ablation and was totally painless. Over the next few days I was a new man, but I realised that the A-Fib would return some

> ❖ *"Unfortunately, he decided to only do the flutter."*
>
> Ken Hungerford

time. It was back less than a week later, but I have never had any more Flutter.

MISERABLE, A-FIB BECOMES UNBEARABLE

By September 2010 (just two months later), the A-Fib had become unbearable, and I was a very miserable old fellow. At times I experienced several episodes a day. They could last several hours or more. And the worst ones felt like I had a maniacal bass drummer hidden away in the chest cavity.

I made another appointment with the EP, Dr. Malcolm Barlow at Lake Macquarie Private Hospital in New South Wales, Australia, for late October 2010, hoping to have a solution presented. He explained that his approach to A-Fib was to use Cryo-ablation, and that it was around 70% successful. The Cryo-ablation is done using an Arctic Front CryoBalloon system. He warned me that there were risks of stroke and damage to the phrenic nerve (that could leave me with breathing problems for a few months).

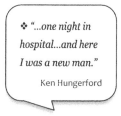

❖ *"...one night in hospital...and here I was a new man."*

Ken Hungerford

After discussing this with my very dear wife, I decided to go ahead with the procedure. A couple of days prior to my admission to the hospital, I had the worst episode I had ever had, almost leaving me in a faint at a local shopping center. I was admitted to the hospital on the 16th of December, 2010, at 6:30 AM.

The procedure started at 9:00 AM, and I was back in the ward at midday, although I don't remember anything before around 3:00 PM that afternoon. I was discharged at 9:30 AM the next morning.

I told my wife that I felt I was a bit of a fraud—one night in hospital, a few hours I cannot remember, absolutely no pain and very little discomfort, and here I was a new man. It feels absolutely marvelous, and I really do feel like a new man.

The only minor crisis I have had since was due to being taken off all the heart medications—warfarin and Sotalol. The EP did not warn me that my pulse rate would increase significantly before settling, and I would also have more Ectopics (heartbeat signals that come from any region of the heart that ordinarily should not produce them). Around four days after taking the last dose of Sotalol, my pulse rate had risen to over 100 bpm, and I was suffering many Ectopics. A visit to the local ER together with a good check-out and call to my EP set my mind at rest.

I don't know whether my success can be generally applied, I can only say how wonderful it has been for me. My life had improved beyond any expectation I ever dared to have!

Physically, I now have energy I have not enjoyed for years, have lost my lethargy and have returned to regular fast walks. Mentally, my wife tells me I'm a far easier person to live with, since I no longer worry about what might happen during the day or night. It is such a relief I just can't explain it in words.

LESSONS LEARNED

I guess I was lucky because I responded so well to cryo-ablation. I know that many people have tried RF ablation, and it has not worked, or they had to have it multiple times. But you just need to keep looking and trying. Otherwise life is just too difficult and unenjoyable.

Best advice: Seek out all the options available.

Ken Hungerford
New South Wales, Australia

Editorial Comments:

Ken was surprised when his A-Fib started post-op. Anyone undergoing cardiac surgery ought to be told there's a 40% chance of developing A-Fib after the surgery.[233] (This risk can often be prevented by prescribing antiarrhythmic meds after surgery.)

Note: Ken's first ablation, for his Atrial Flutter, was performed in the right atrium, and later a second ablation for his A-Fib was performed in his left atrium. Current research indicates that an ablation in the right atrium for Atrial Flutter has little chance of also curing A-Fib (which generally comes from the left atrium).[234] To avoid having to do two separate ablation procedures, most centers now do both Atrial Flutter and A-Fib ablations at the same time.

With 'Silent' A-Fib Decides on Watchman Device to Ditch the Drugs

Tom has Silent A-Fib (A-Fib with few noticeable symptoms) and had been on Coumadin for six years to address the associated risk of clots and A-Fib stroke. Then, out of the blue, a phone call offered him an alternative to the meds and monthly blood tests.

I HAD A SUDDEN, severe A-Fib attack in 2001. It was painful, pounding and felt like a heart attack. But after an injection of medicine in the ER, I went back into normal sinus rhythm within a minute. But about eight weeks later I developed A-Fib again. An EKG at Massachusetts General Hospital confirmed that I did have so-called "permanent" A-Fib.

Tom Paxman
Boston, MA, USA

ON COUMADIN FOR SIX YEARS

I was on Coumadin (warfarin), and understandably worried about the risk of blood clots and stroke while in A-Fib. But it was difficult keeping the proper blood levels [AN INR BETWEEN 2 AND 3] using the blood thinner. I had to take monthly blood draws for six years which were a real nuisance.

By that time I was always in A-Fib (Persistent Long-standing A-Fib). The steroid inhaler I use makes my skin very thin. I bruise easily.

The blood thinning effects of Coumadin make me even more susceptible to bruising and bleeding.

❖ *"I had to take monthly blood draws for six years which were a real nuisance."*

Tom Paxman

A-FIB NOT SYMPTOMATIC—DECIDED AGAINST A PVI PROCEDURE

I decided against having a Pulmonary Vein Isolation procedure or surgery to fix my persistent A-Fib. I was 70 years old, and my A-Fib was *not* symptomatic. I had also been battling Chronic Obstructive Pulmonary Disease (COPD) for many years and had degenerative disc disease.

I was told I might be a good candidate for a Pulmonary Vein Isolation procedure, but I declined. My own feeling was the less intervention or intrusion in your body you can avoid, the better off you are. Some things are obviously necessary, but this was kind of optional. I thought I'll just keep up with the blood testing once a month, even though it was a huge pain. I didn't know of any other alternative.

WATCHMAN DEVICE OPTION

Then in 2009, Dr. Moussa Mansour of Mass. General called me to introduce himself and describe a new option to possibly replace Coumadin called the Watchman device. After extensive discussion with my doctor, I decided to have the Watchman device installed to close off the Left Atrial Appendage (LAA) where 90%–95% of A-Fib blood clots come from.

Though like Coumadin it wouldn't be an absolute guarantee of preventing an A-Fib stroke and I'd still be in A-Fib, the Watchman device would enable me to get off of Coumadin. I had the Watchman device installed in late 2009.

❖ *"I'd still be in A-Fib, (but) the Watchman device would enable me to get off of Coumadin."*

Tom Paxman

Before installing the Watchman device, they inserted a tube down my esophagus to see if I had any clots, and to get a closer picture of my heart. This test caused a moderate sore throat. (If they had found any clots, they would first dissolve them with additional blood thinners before installing the Watchman device.)

In a follow-up exam a year after the Watchman device was installed, the same test was repeated to make sure there was a perfect fit and that the LAA was completely closed off.

I don't feel any different. Fortunately, I don't take any blood thinners and don't have to make those monthly trips to the lab to have blood drawn which was a real nuisance. In other respects I am now normal. I could go for an ablation. But I figure I'd better be happy with ¾ of a loaf rather than try to get the whole loaf. It isn't like I'm 45 or 50 and have a lot of years left.

I don't feel the Watchman device interferes with my life. I have no idea it's in there. I don't have to worry about it. I got rid of the blood clot ordeal. Nothing else is different, except that I now have some "peace of mind."

I've since joined a new local fitness gym because I was quite out of shape, primarily due to the limitations of COPD and four lumbar disc operations. Since then, I am much stronger, etc. and now look forward to my gym workouts. The point is, A-Fib and the Watchman have not interfered with or restricted my lifestyle at all.

LESSONS LEARNED

Ideally, try ablations. And if that fails, do this Watchman procedure which has a very high rate of success.

I wish we knew what causes A-Fib so we could take steps to avoid it. I don't believe it's hereditary. [SEE EDITORIAL COMMENTS BELOW.] And we don't really know what the possible causes are. The first attack is very scary—I thought I was having a heart attack.

A-Fib victims need to realize that A-Fib is not a "killer disease" but simply a heart condition that should be treated and monitored. And the only worry is about blood clots forming which can/will cause stroke. My type of A-Fib [ASYMPTOMATIC] is more of a nuisance as long as it is under control. Nevertheless, the chance of stroke is a legitimate concern, which is why the Watchman Device is so valuable in lessening or fully preventing stroke.

I still have A-Fib, but the Watchman device has reduced the chance of stroke by about 90-95%, I believe. Even though I am in A-Fib all the time, I simply don't worry about A-Fib anymore.

Tom Paxman
Boston, Mass. USA

Editorial Comments:

Tom Paxman's A-Fib was asymptomatic, i.e., he had no noticeable symptoms. This was a major factor in his declining a catheter ablation. (Many centers will not do an ablation if a patient has no or few symptoms.)

But while his Atrial Fibrillation did not manifest symptoms, he was still at risk for A-Fib blood clots and stroke. The Watchman device addressed his risk of stroke and eliminated the need for blood thinners and the associated monthly monitoring tests as well.

Use of a Watchman device or other occlusion devices does not guarantee you will not have an A-Fib stroke. It does, however, give patients like Tom a welcome alternative to taking blood thinners. (But keep in mind, taking a blood thinner, like warfarin, is also not a guarantee you will not have an A-Fib stroke. It reduces the risk of stroke by 60% to 70%.[235] That still leaves a significant chance of an A-Fib stroke.)

Is A-Fib hereditary? While Tom has his doubts, research indicates an individual's risk of Atrial Fibrillation increases 40% if a first-degree relative (parent or sibling) has Atrial Fibrillation.[236] This is independent of research that has identified four rare genetic variants known to influence A-Fib risk.[237] It's possible that people with A-Fib have a genetic predisposition not yet identified by current research.[238]

Annoying A-Fib Symptoms Worsen & Turn Critical With Threat of Sick Sinus Syndrome

For years Joy's A-Fib symptoms were mostly annoying. In 2010 they worsened into near-fainting episodes. Fear of an A-Fib episode overshadowed activities she once enjoyed with her teenage daughter. On the verge of developing sick sinus syndrome, she had a decision to make.

FOR THE PAST FIVE YEARS, I've had occasional A-Fib episodes. I was highly symptomatic, but typically would self-convert within two-three hours with no lingering side effects other than those similar to insomnia. So A-Fib didn't really have a significant impact on my life. My cardiologist would periodically give me a Holter monitor in hopes of catching an episode on it, but for four years we were unsuccessful with our timing.

Joy Gray and daughter
Manchester, New
Hampshire, USA

ER VISITS AND MAJOR BLOOD PRESSURE DROP

Summer 2010, I started having longer, more intense episodes and in July I had an episode that did not self-convert. I went to the Emergency Room in the morning and was loaded up on the normal drugs (Lovenox and Cardizem) and then admitted as an outpatient to await a cardioversion the next morning. They gave me a load-in dosage of Flecanide at dinner time. I converted back to Sinus Rhythm shortly after — too soon for it to have been because of the Flecanide, according to my EP. About an hour after converting, my blood pressure dropped. I began to feel light-headed even though I was lying slightly elevated in a hospital bed. My face became numb; the nurses elevated my feet to bring my blood pressure back up.

I went home the next evening, still on the Flecanide. I lasted three days on the Flecanide before I was back to the ER, this time with symptomatic bradycardia. Every time I would doze off to sleep, my heart rate would drop into the 30s with significant PVCs which would wake me up. I hadn't slept in three nights and was absolutely miserable. The EP pulled me off the Flecanide with a follow up appointment scheduled about a month later.

❖ *"A catheter ablation was out of the question as I have an Amplatzer device."*

Joy Gray

EP SUGGESTS MINI-MAZE

At this time, he first suggested the Mini-Maze as he did not feel I was a good candidate for anti-arrhythmic medications. A catheter ablation was out of the question as I have an Amplatzer device between my Atria that was used to close my Atrial Septal Defect. While there have been a few (very few) catheter ablations done on patients with this device, neither my EP nor I felt that I was a good candidate for this still experimental procedure. At that time I opted to take a wait and see approach as I had lived with this for at least five years without too much disruption in my life.

TOUGHING IT OUT AT HOME, MORE BLOOD PRESSURE DROPS

I had a few more mild episodes in the fall, but always self-converted quickly. In January [2011], I had another longer episode, and decided to try to tough it out at home. I came very close to passing out a few minutes after converting, and was miserable the rest of the day.

About three weeks later I had yet another episode. I was on my way to my doctor's office to await cardioversion when I converted. We went into the office to have an EKG to confirm that I had actually converted, and in the process of getting the results, my blood pressure once again plummeted and I almost blacked out. The cardiologist rushed me to the Emergency Room, where I basically rested for a couple of hours before they sent me home.

> ❖ "...my blood pressure once again plummeted and I almost blacked out."
>
> Joy Gray

A-FIB INTOLERABLE AND DISRUPTIVE OF FAMILY LIFE

Up until January 2011, my symptoms, while annoying, were not really disrupting my life. But once I started having the near-fainting episodes, A-Fib became very disruptive. I became much more cautious about anything that might trigger an episode and started worrying about having an episode the night before any family event, making it difficult to look forward to these events. I did have a few more episodes and found that I could no longer just go on with my life afterward – I needed at least 24 hours of rest after an A-Fib episode to return to any degree of normalcy.

Activities that I once enjoyed with my 13 year old daughter became difficult because of the fear of an A-Fib episode—who would drive us home if I went into A-Fib two hours away? Would we have to call my husband at work and have him come pick us up?

SAYS "NO" TO A LIFETIME OF DRUGS

My EP, Dr. Daniel Philbin of New England Heart Institute, said that he believed I was developing sick sinus syndrome, and once again recommended the Mini-Maze. And this time I was more inclined to agree. The other option was to have a pacemaker inserted and try some of the other anti-arrhythmic drugs. My EP still didn't feel that I was a good candidate for tolerating the drugs, and I agreed with him. At 46, a lifetime of drugs that are as bad as the disease had no appeal.

> ❖ "At 46, a lifetime of drugs that are as bad as the disease had no appeal."
>
> Joy Gray

There was one more factor to consider in my case— several years earlier I had been diagnosed with a mild fibrinogen deficiency (a very rare inherited blood coagulation disorder), which impacts how my blood clots. This might cause difficulty with Coumadin regulation in the future (if I needed anticoagulation therapy), and I wasn't eager to find out if I could tolerate Coumadin or not. The Mini-Maze would almost certainly allow me to delay the need for Coumadin therapy, or maybe avoid it altogether.

I contacted the surgeon recommended by Dr. Philbin along with two other surgeons I had found through my own research. I should mention that I really like and trust Dr. Philbin, and he encouraged me to contact a couple of other well-known surgeons prior to making my final decision so that I could be comfortable that I had made the best decision for myself. Ultimately, after speaking to each surgeon, I found I was most comfortable with the surgeon my EP recommended, Dr. Ralph Damiano, Jr. of Barnes-Jewish Hospital and Washington University Medical Center in St. Louis, Missouri.

TRAVEL TO ST. LOUIS AND PRE-OP TESTING

We arrived in St. Louis by air on July 4, and checked into our hotel. I had blood work, an echocardiogram, and a consult visit scheduled for the morning of July 5, with the procedure scheduled for July 7.

> ❖ *"...during the night I was awakened by the nursing staff because my heart rate had dropped into the 30s."*
>
> Joy Gray

After the consult I was admitted to Barnes-Jewish Hospital for a heart catheterization to check for any blockages and to have a hematology consult to address the fibrinogen issue.

They also had the anesthesiologist come in to speak with me about what would happen prior to, during, and after the mini-maze procedure. My heart rate was in the low 40s when I was admitted, and at one point during the night I was awakened by the nursing staff because my heart rate had dropped into the 30s.

THE MINI-MAZE AND RECOVERY

I went into the operating room around 1 PM and woke up in ICU for recovery before 6 PM. At first I was doing very well but then my left side started experiencing strong muscle spasms in my lower back and shoulder. It was determined I needed something stronger than Percocet for the pain. And as soon as I received that, I rested comfortably.

The painkillers kept me a bit hazy, so all I am certain of is that sometime the next afternoon I was moved to the cardiac floor from ICU.

From there my recovery went very well. I was able to get out of bed and walk without assistance by the third day after the procedure, and had we been nearer home, could have likely gone home the fourth day.

Because of my prior intolerance for antiarrhythmics and the fibrinogen deficiency, the initial decision was to have me leave the hospital only on the medications I came in with – a beta blocker and aspirin.

A-FIB RETURNS

The sixth day after my procedure I was dressed and ready to leave the hospital when I felt my heart rhythm change to A-Fib. I was re-attached to cardiac monitoring, which confirmed I was in either A-Fib or Flutter with a heart rate over 150. I was readmitted to the hospital without ever making it out the door.

> ❖ *"I was readmitted to the hospital without ever making it out the door."*
>
> Joy Gray

For the next 24 hours I was in and out of A-Fib,

with a heart rate that ranged from 40 to 190. At one point to bring my heart rate down I was given an IV injection of beta blocker, and my heart rate went to the 30s. There was some discussion of a pacemaker so that I could tolerate higher dosages of rate control medicine, but there was also a good deal of resistance to that idea.

At that point, I really didn't care what they did as long as they did something. I was now having more A-Fib/Flutter than I had ever had prior to the procedure.

GOING HOME WITH AMIODARONE AND COUMADIN

Eight days after the procedure, I was given a heparin IV and started on Coumadin. In addition, I was started on a load-in dose of amiodarone.

I remained in the hospital another week as a "Coumadin hostage" because my INR wasn't high enough to be released, and I was still in and out of A-Fib at least twice a day. Finally, on the day doctors were ready to switch me to Pradaxa so I could go home, my INR topped 2.0 for the first time. I left the hospital that afternoon, and went straight to the airport and had a thankfully uneventful flight home.

RECOVERY AT HOME

My recovery at home has gone well. I had one instance of A-Fib with rates in the 120s the first day I was home, while the visiting nurse was at our house. That was sixteen days after the procedure and eight days after my first dose of amiodarone. I had one more very brief episode three days later and have been A-Fib free since then. I am now 37 days post procedure.

> ❖ *"I have 11 incisions not including the groin incision for the heart cath."*
>
> Joy Gray

I have 11 incisions not including the groin incision for the heart cath. While healing, the incisions are uncomfortable, but not truly painful. As I become more active each day, I tend to stretch them a bit more – so it feels more like overworked muscles than pain. I occasionally take a Tylenol when I overdo it a bit; I am not one who tolerates pain well.

The more annoying recovery issues I've had include that the breathing tube irritated my throat significantly, and I had significant laryngitis and throat issues for almost a month. The oxygen given after the procedure irritated my nose, triggering almost constant nosebleeds (pre-Coumadin). Finally my PCP [PREFERRED CARE PHYSICIAN] cauterized two spots in my nose to stem the bleeding.

> ❖ *"I now have an Atri-Clip to occlude the left atrial appendage."*
>
> Joy Gray

As part of the procedure, I now have an AtriClip[239] to occlude the left atrial appendage (the AtriClip is an alternative to suture or staples for closing off the LAA). I have not noted any side effects from this. I was expecting to have to monitor my fluid intake, but thus far if anything I have found myself more thirsty than normal. I try to keep water with me at all times.

I have been fortunate enough to have a relatively stable INR on Coumadin, and not to have any apparent side effects from the amiodarone. I was able to drive

30 days after the procedure, and feel quite comfortable driving except for some muscle soreness.

NORMAL SINUS RHYTHM!

My resting heart rate now ranges from this high 50s to the 70s – a welcome change from the 40s before the procedure. Dr. Philbin states that this is a result of the "work" done during the Mini-Maze.

I also no longer suffer from the constant PVCs/PACs that I experienced prior to the procedure, but I have been warned that those will likely return after I come off the amiodarone. My blood pressure is running a bit on the low side in the mornings, but I've learned to live with that by being cautious not to make sudden movements or position changes.

For now, I'm enjoying a normal sinus rhythm for the first time in six years with no PVCs/PACs and no bradycardia, and no A-Fib, too!

> ❖ *"If you aren't comfortable with your first doctor—find another."*
>
> Joy Gray

LESSONS LEARNED

Educate yourself about your condition. Find an EP you are comfortable with as soon as possible—if you aren't comfortable with your first doctor, find another. You need a medical professional you can trust to provide sound treatment advice.

A-Fib tends to be a progressive disease, so taking an aggressive approach to treatment early on may be your best option.

Realize that there are others who have been through this, find them, and use them as part of your support system [SEE APPENDIX B FOR ONLINE SUPPORT GROUPS].

Also realize that A-Fib is not "one size fits all."

In various online support groups some people push (or seem to push) one treatment/procedure/surgeon over another. This doesn't mean that if you select a different alternative, you are wrong. Each of us has unique circumstances that shape our decisions. Most of the support group members just hope your treatment works for you.

Joy Gray
Manchester, New Hampshire, USA

Editorial Comments:
To close off her Left Atrial Appendage (LAA), Joy's surgeon implanted an AtriClip. Working from outside the heart and the LAA, the rectangular-shaped device is positioned around the LAA, then closed like a clamp, blocking the flow of blood into and out of the LAA. It's an alternative to the use of sutures or staples. The AtriClip by AtriCure has a similar function as the Atritech Watchman device, a catheter delivered device positioned from inside the heart at the opening of the LAA.

Being only 46 years old, Joy didn't want to spend the rest of her life on drugs. She couldn't have a catheter ablation, because an Amplatzer device was previously installed to plug a hole in her septum. A Mini Maze was her best and probably her only option.

It's unfortunate that Joy's A-Fib returned after her surgery, and that she had to be put on amiodarone and Coumadin. Amiodarone (a toxic med not intended for long term use) is an effective antiarrhythmic that may help her heart get used to beating normally. Since her Left Atrial Appendage was closed off, she may be able to stop the Coumadin, as well.

As Joy's story demonstrates, maze surgeries (and catheter ablations too) aren't always unqualified successes. But Joy has made it through the worst part, and her quality of life is much improved. Let's hope she remains A-Fib free.

Misdiagnosed as Anxiety, Later Found A-Fib Cure Through a Clinical Trial

Terry was seeing a therapist because he thought his "attacks" were caused by anxiety; after his A-Fib diagnosis, many drug therapies followed. His cure came in 2007 from a clinical trial for CryoBalloon ablation.

I HAD A CRYOBALLOON ABLATION at Massachusetts General Hospital by Dr. Vivek Reddy on July 11, 2007. I participated in the pivotal STOP A-Fib Trial (Sustained Treatment of Paroxysmal Atrial Fibrillation) using Pulmonary Vein Isolation. Dr. Reddy also used the CryoCath Freezor Max catheter to treat my atrial flutter.

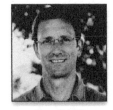

I've benefited greatly from the wise counsel on A-Fib.com and hope my story will be helpful to others. I was diagnosed with A-Fib at age 43. Once I knew what A-Fib felt like, I could see that I had been having events

Terry DeWitt
Massachusetts, USA

since the late 1990s and maybe earlier. I would often wake up in the middle of the night short of breath and had several episodes during athletic activities as well.

THOUGHT SYMPTOMS WERE ANXIETY OR ASTHMA

Prior to my diagnosis I had thought these events were anxiety or asthma attacks. Consequently, I was seeing a therapist and had been on Klonopin (anxiety medication) for four years. I also was on maintenance doses of Flovent (asthma medication) which I took daily, and carried another inhaler for use during my attacks.

> ❖ *"Prior to my diagnosis I had thought these events were anxiety or asthma attacks. Consequently, I was seeing a therapist..."*
>
> Terry DeWitt

I have been an avid endurance athlete since I rowed crew at Harvard. In 2001, I participated for the second time in the Canadian Cross-country Ski Marathon which is 100 miles over two days, the longest cross-country skiing event in the world. The first day was canceled due to high winds. Early the next morning while taking the bus to the start for the second day, I noticed that my heart rate monitor read 120 bpm just sitting there on the bus. "Boy, am I excited about this race!" I said to myself. Well, once the race started I knew differently! Everyone passed me. I must have fallen down 15 times due to weakness in my legs.

Thinking my shortness of breath was due to asthma or lack of training, I kept going eventually and painfully finishing the 50 mile day. It never occurred to me it could be my heart!

A year later I was finally diagnosed. Initially no medication was prescribed as I went through the battery of tests: Holter monitor, chemical stress test, and echocardiogram. Then one episode put me in the emergency room, and I was put on Norpace.

Following several A-Fib episodes, I was put on Pindolol, and the Norpace was replaced by Flecainide. The medication succeeded in stopping my A-Fib, but I had difficulty tolerating the side effects: shortness of breath, dizziness, low energy, heavy legs, and night sweats, yuck!

While all this was going on, I enrolled myself in the Cardiac Wellness Program at Dr. Herb Benson's Mind Body Medical Institute to focus on heart health via meditation, relaxation, nutrition, and light exercise. Their program helped me, but was more focused on heart disease than arrhythmia. At this point I limited myself to walking on a treadmill a half hour a day at eight degrees tilt and lifting moderate weights at 15 reps twice a week. I meditated 20 minutes a day.

> ❖ *"The medication succeeded in stopping my A-Fib, but I had difficulty tolerating the side effects: shortness of breath, dizziness, low energy, heavy legs, and night sweats, yuck!"*
>
> Terry DeWitt

In December, I replaced the Pindolol with Metoprolol to no large improvement in side effects. In the following February, I replaced the Metoprolol with Cartia XT and saw some side effect improvement but also started having A-Fib events again. In early March, I replaced the Flecainide with Rythmol and saw additional side effect improvements, but also started having A-Fib episodes more often and of longer duration.

WITH MORE AND LONGER EPISODES CONSIDERS ABLATION

I had been considering having an ablation but wanted to try out all my chemical options first. I knew I could continue on medication for several years, but my quality of life was definitely suffering. I was having difficulty concentrating at work, and all I wanted to do was sit in front of the TV at home. I was having episodes every week or two, and I was concerned about the remodeling of my heart. I decided this had to change and that, although it had risks, ablation was a route I had to try. It seemed I would need an ablation sooner or later; and sooner, when my heart was still strong and I was still paroxysmal, seemed better.

I chose Dr. Vivek Reddy at MGH [MASSACHUSETTS GENERAL HOSPITAL] as the best guy in New England. My insurance would only cover me if I stayed in New England. We set a date for the procedure.

CRYOABLATION CLINICAL TRIAL AT MASS GENERAL

Then I got a call from him offering me a chance to participate in a clinical trial for Cryoablation. The trial was such that, if I agreed to participate, I would have a 2/3 chance of getting the Cryoablation procedure immediately. I had a 1/3 chance of being placed in the control group and would have to take medications for six more months, then I could have the Cryoablation.

I was naturally concerned about participating in a clinical trial. Ablations have enough risk as it is. I was cautious about adding more. But the more I learned about Cryo, the more I realized that it was theoretically safer than radio frequency energy. Cryo does less damage to tissue than RF and consequently is less likely to create problems like esophageal fistula, pulmonary vein stenosis, stroke, etc. And rather than using a pencil type catheter, in Cryo you can use a balloon catheter which theoretically can produce a more uniform ablation.

While the CryoCath Arctic Front balloon catheter is approved in Europe, it was not yet approved in the US. Dr. Reddy was one of two doctors in the country to perform the first stage of the trial, with 20 patients each. Success rate with no medication was about 75%, which is comparable to RF ablation. Dr. Reddy had also performed another 20 in Eastern Europe. He had also demonstrated a Cryoablation at the Boston Atrial Fibrillation Symposium.

Because of the success of the initial trial, the FDA approved the second "pivotal trial" of some 200 patients in many more centers across the country. This trial would use the next generation CryoCath Arctic Front balloon catheter with two balloon sizes instead of one and a more flexible sheath.

PARTICIPATES IN CLINICAL TRIAL

When I spoke with Dr. Reddy about my participation in the trial, he said I could expect a comparable success rate to RF, but with less risk. I asked him if it was his family member who had the choice, what would he do? He said he would choose the Cryo, even if he had to wait the six months extra to get it. He was convinced it was safer due to the reduced tissue damage. The real question according to him was whether the Cryo lesions would be effective for as long as RF lesions. Since this is new, no one knows the answer to that yet.

> ❖ *"The real question according to Dr. Reddy was whether the Cryo lesions would be effective for as long as RF lesions."*
>
> Terry DeWitt

Needless to say I decided to do the Cryo, constantly reading all I could to find a reason not to believe my doctor. Beyond the obvious conflict of interest, everything I read said that Cryo had the most promise of being the next generation technique for A-Fib ablation, because it was likely to be safer. And I knew I had the most experienced Cryo guy in the country as my doctor.

Just before my procedure, CryoCath published an article covering a study of over 300 Cryoablations presented at the European Society of Cardiology (Europace) Conference in Lisbon. They reported an 84% success rate with paroxysmal patients. They also reported a 7.5% incident of phrenic nerve injury, which is high; although all of them resolved on their own in less than a year. (The phrenic nerve helps the diaphragm expand so you can take air into your lungs.) The article noted that no esophageal fistula or pulmonary vein stenosis was reported (potential risks of RF ablations).

MY CRYOBALLOON ABLATION PROCEDURE

My procedure took place on July 11, 2007. Due to unrelated back pain which made it painful for me to lie flat, I had general anesthesia rather than the normal sedation. As a result, I can't tell you much about the procedure experience since I was asleep. One thing I do know was that it took a long time, due to the study protocols. I was put under around 8 AM and woke up around 3:30 PM for a total time of about 7 ½ hours.

Following the procedure I was told that they successfully isolated the pulmonary veins but that there was some phrenic nerve damage. Apparently they make you hiccup to be sure the phrenic nerve is not harmed. When I stopped hiccupping, they immediately stopped ablating. I resumed hiccupping about ten minutes later. Upon examination, I was taking air into both lungs, but the chest X-ray did show one side of my diaphragm noticeably higher than the left. I was told this almost always resolves within a year, and they would follow this closely.

RECOVERY: AFTER MY PROCEDURE

During recovery in the hospital the same day and next day, I definitely felt discomfort in my chest—kind of a burning and heaviness that was worse when I lay down. I had no noticeable trouble breathing at all. I also noticed a sore throat that made it difficult to eat anything but soft foods.

I went home on schedule the day after the procedure. Two days later I called my doctor as he instructed because I was still having some chest pain and wanted pain medication. When I mentioned I was still having pain when swallowing food, he decided to re-admit me to be extra sure there was no damage to my esophagus (scary!). He told me he was very sure all was fine but wanted to be safe. First I had a chest CT scan that didn't show anything definitive about my esophagus, but did show moderate fluid around my heart and a bit of fluid also in my lungs.

> ❖ *"...he decided to re-admit me to be extra sure there was no damage to my esophagus (scary!)."*
>
> Terry DeWitt

Apparently no big deal other than to monitor (I had no fever). The next day they put a camera down my throat under sedation and discovered that I had an infection which could be treated with an antibiotic. Apparently the instruments they put down your throat with anesthesia had disrupted an infection already brewing, or perhaps created one. Either way it was easily treated, to my relief.

MY LIFE IS BACK!

I was very happy to have emerged relatively unscathed from the procedure, and I have been in sinus rhythm steadily since. I have great faith in Dr. Reddy and feel I was well served under his care.

At my one month check-up in August 2007, the phrenic nerve damage had completely resolved. Dr. Reddy discontinued Rythmol at that appointment and my Cartia XT two weeks later. Once I stopped taking those medications, I felt my energy returning, my head clearing up, and most of the side effects I'd been experiencing vanished. The next month or so were spent taking half hour walks at lunch and slowly increasing my activity level. I had some persistent discomfort in my chest, particularly upon exertion, that seemed to be due to some lingering inflammation around my heart. A few days of Motrin cleared that up.

> ❖ *"Once I stopped taking those medications, I felt my energy returning, my head clearing up...."*
>
> Terry DeWitt

I worked up to about 30 minutes of aerobic exercise five days a week at a heart rate of about 125 bpm. I added weights (high reps) two or three times a week for about 20 minutes. This level of activity seemed about right without pushing it too hard.

Following two holters two weeks apart, I was allowed to stop taking Coumadin. I was then completely off all of my meds and feeling better than I had in a long time. I was very glad I pursued the Cryoablation.

Since that time, the FDA CryoBalloon trial concluded; In December 2010 the FDA approved use of the CryoBalloon catheter in the U.S. for pulmonary vein ablations. It is now almost four years since I participated in the pivotal STOP A-Fib Trial with Dr. Vivek Reddy and Massachusetts General Hospital.

I am very happy to report that I have not had a single A-Fib event since my procedure.

I now exercise one to 1 ½ hours per day, six days per week and feel great. I honestly feel as good as I did before all the A-Fib episodes started. This summer I brought my eight-year-old daughter up Mt. Adams, the second tallest mountain in New England. I'm truly as good as new. Well, maybe a few years older!

In speaking with Dr. Jeremy Ruskin, head of the program at Mass General (Dr. Vivek Reddy is now at Mount Sinai in NY), the patients that participated in the CryoBalloon trial have responded particularly well, with relatively low relapse [recurrence] and good recovery.

> ❖ *"I went undiagnosed for about 5 years. Primary care physicians don't consider that young people can get A-Fib."*
>
> Terry DeWitt

LESSONS LEARNED

I wish I had known that all my shortness of breath and feeling of anxiety were due to my heart and A-Fib [AND NOT ANXIETY OR ASTHMA AS HE HAD SPECULATED].

I went undiagnosed for about five years. Primary care physicians don't consider that young people can get A-Fib, and don't know how to test for it. (I was given a stress test rather than a Holter monitor.)

I recommend that everyone consider the CryoBalloon, in addition to radio frequency for their catheter ablation. Generally, it is safer and has as good or better outcome. I had great success, and Mass General is pleased with the results their Cryo patients are having. But I would also suggest finding a doctor who has significant experience using the CryoBalloon. A list of doctors who participated in the STOP A-Fib trial should be available online.

Best Advice: Spend the time to find the best Electrophysiologist (arrhythmia specialist) you can find. It makes a big difference in treatment and in the success of the ablation procedure.

Terry DeWitt
Massachusetts, USA

Editorial Comments:

Prior to his A-Fib diagnosis, Terry thought his "events" were anxiety or asthma attacks. Misdiagnosis happens. Other medical conditions can mimic an arrhythmia. Stress and anxiety can cause heart palpitations, rapid heartbeat and shortness of breath pointing to Hyperventilation or Chronic Panic Disorder (CPD). A standard workup may have eliminated these causes. Certainly, an ECG during one of his "events" would have revealed his Atrial Fibrillation earlier.

Terry's procedure was part of a FDA clinical trial. In December 2010, the FDA approved use of the CryoBalloon catheter in the U.S. for pulmonary vein ablations. A major medical advance in the treatment of A-Fib, many centers now offer CryoBalloon ablation. It is faster and easier for doctors to perform, and appears safer for patients.

During his 2007 procedure, Terry incurred short-term damage to his Phrenic Nerve (often found near the Right Superior Pulmonary Vein). Nowadays doctors take specific precautions to protect the nerve. During CryoBalloon ablations, doctors routinely "stimulate" and monitor the nerve. If they see that the Cryo energy is affecting it, they stop ablating in that area and let the Phrenic Nerve "defrost" and return to normal. Today, damage to the Phrenic Nerve is much less of a problem.

Binge Drinking Leads to Chronic A-Fib, Amiodarone Damages Eyesight

Kris was admitted for double pneumonia when they discovered Atrial Fibrillation. She tells how her A-Fib was brought on by a combination of alcohol, stress, bacterial pneumonia and over-the-counter cold medications.

IN NOVEMBER OF 2008 I was admitted to the hospital with double pneumonia. I also had an excessively fast heartbeat that averaged 140 beats per minute. My GP tried different meds to slow the beat, but my heart would not go below 90 beats per minute. I was in a rural country hospital that housed an outreach clinic for the University of Iowa Cardiovascular Unit.

I was fortunate that the outreach clinic's heart specialist took over my case. He ordered an EKG which showed that I had Atrial Fibrillation. I remember thinking this is not possible for me to have

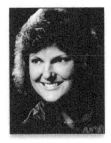

Kris, Iowa, USA

a heart condition! I am barely over 50—this can't be happening to me! But it was. I was transported by ambulance to the University of Iowa Cardiovascular Unit within six hours of being diagnosed with A-Fib.

> ❖ *"Each had a different opinion, but none of them would tell me what would happen next."*
>
> Kris

The next five days I spent in the U of Iowa Hospital going through various tests which included a cardiac catheterization to see if I had a blood clot or blockage of the heart. The doctors performed an endoscopic (EGD) test where they insert a flexible tube outfitted with a light and camera down the throat to have a look for abnormalities.

The University is a teaching college, so I had a staff of specialists, fellows and doctors coming in to visit me. Each had a different opinion, but none of them would tell me what would happen next. I learned that by being persistent I could generally find one doctor who would answer my questions giving the explanations that I needed.

ELECTRICAL CARDIOVERSION

I was scheduled for a cardio convert on November 23rd. The convert successfully put my heart back into sinus rhythm. The procedure was performed in the afternoon, and I was immediately released to go home. I didn't understand why I could go home so quickly after I had just spent five days in the cardiac unit. I was told there was nothing more that could be done. We had to wait to see if the heart would heal and stay in sinus rhythm.

I was also given an array of medicine: lisinopral (blood pressure med that works through the kidneys), metoprolol (blood pressure med that works on the heart muscle), furosemide (fluid med or 'water pill' that is used to reduce fluid retention), Coumadin (warfarin–a blood thinner), digoxin (used to regulate the heart) and omerprazole (Prilosec–to keep me from getting nausea so that I could take the other meds). I wasn't told much about side effects of the meds. I found out more about side effects of the meds from the pharmacists than I did from the medical team at the hospital. I do experience fairly interesting side effects from meds, so I need to know all I can about meds that I am taking.

BACK IN A-FIB

By the 19th of December my heart was back in A-Fib. I felt I had a death sentence even though I was told by doctors and nurses that "If you have to have a heart condition, A-Fib is the one to have. It is more of an inconvenience than life threatening." This is not exactly what a person going through depression, weight loss, fatigue and with an irregular heart wants to hear. The best I got was to go on another med: amiodarone—which slows the heart by relaxing the heart muscle. The plan was to determine what was causing my A-Fib and schedule another cardio-convert after my INR blood level tested between 2 and 3 for three weeks straight, to ensure that a blood clot wouldn't form.

ADMITTING TO ALCOHOL ADDICTION

One of the most difficult things that I had to admit to was to tell my doctor that I drank alcohol excessively. I have an addictive behavior disorder – which is another story – and most people would consider me an alcoholic. Binge drinking is one of the top five causes of A-Fib. My A-Fib was brought on by a combination of alcohol, stress, bacterial pneumonia and over the counter cold medications. I could have prevented my A-Fib by not drinking alcohol in excess, but most A-Fib can't be prevented.

> ❖ "One of the most difficult things that I had to admit to was to tell my doctor that I drank alcohol excessively."
>
> Kris

BACK IN EMERGENCY ROOM

I proceeded to have the scariest six weeks of my life waiting for the INR level to stabilize to have my second cardio-convert. My heart became totally erratic. Light headedness usually happened within ½ hour of taking the meds. I would wake up in the middle of the night with a bizarre sensation and butterflies in my stomach. Sometimes all I could do was to walk in order to work the heart muscle so that I would feel better.

I ended up in the emergency room one evening because my heartbeat totally flipped out and my blood pressure crashed. Nothing out of the ordinary was found after the EKG was read. I was given an anti-anxiety med with script to fill and sent home. I tried to reach the heart specialist through his nurse. I described my symptoms but was told that I had to have blood pressure readings to give to the doctor before anything could be done. I should have pushed harder. It seems that the combination of digoxin and amiodarone was too much for me.

SUCCESSFUL ELECTRICAL CARDIOVERSION!

Finally the INR stabilized for three weeks, so another cardio convert was performed. My doctor told my sister that he expected my heart to be back in A-Fib within six months. But I wasn't told this until a year and half later. I had a small miracle when my heart stayed in sinus rhythm for one and a half years. I became my doctor's 'successful project'.

AMIODARONE DAMAGES EYESIGHT, BUT NOT PERMANENTLY

Shortly after the second cardio convert, I began to have difficulty focusing, so I made an appointment to have my eyes checked. I thought it was time to get stronger contact lenses. My optometrist was concerned when he discovered I was taking amiodarone.

> ❖ *"...one of the side effects of amiodarone was a chemical buildup on the retina that could eventually damage eyesight."*
>
> Kris

He said that one of the side effects of amiodarone was a chemical buildup on the retina that could eventually damage eyesight. But my medical doctor assured me that I would not be on the amiodarone long enough to cause lasting adverse side effects. I stopped taking the amiodarone in June of 2009. Within 3 ½ months my eyesight improved. I guess that weak eyesight versus an arrhythmia is the lesser of two evils.

IN CHRONIC A-FIB

In June of 2010 I went for my checkup only to be told that I was in A-Fib again. I had guessed that the arrhythmia had just happened. I was outside on a hot humid day doing very physical labor that caused an increase of adrenaline and stress. My heart went back into A-Fib. The decision was to wait three to four months to see if my heart would revert to sinus rhythm on its own. It didn't. I had chronic (i.e. Long-standing Persistent) A-Fib. I would have good days and bad days. I was constantly fatigued. I had palpitations almost every day. I just didn't feel well. It showed in my personality.

I did not consider this a quality life.

DECIDING ON AN ABLATION

In September of 2010 my doctor told me I would need to make a decision on how to treat the A-Fib. Three different treatments have shown success. The first was to control the rhythm with meds. I was tired of fighting the med side effects. I also didn't feel that meds were successfully controlling my A-Fib. The second was to have another cardio-convert. But studies are showing that cardio-converts are only successful for a short period. The third treatment is an ablation. It was scary thinking about a doctor going up a vein at the groin to 'burn' part of your heart to change the electrical signals to obtain sinus rhythm.

> ❖ *"It was scary thinking about a doctor going up a vein at the groin to 'burn' part of your heart."*
>
> Kris

I wanted to fix or cure the A-Fib; so an appointment was made for a preliminary consultation with Dr. Alexander Mazur, an ablation specialist at the University of Iowa Cardiovascular Clinic. Sure, I considered going for a second opinion. But I couldn't see increasing the time I was in A-Fib to find another medical facility for a consultation.

So I researched the U of I specialist that would perform the ablation. I found that he had been performing ablation procedures first in Europe and then the United States for over ten years. He was brought to the U of I as a teacher and to help expand the Cardiovascular Clinic's ability to treat arrhythmias. I was comfortable – besides I was very impatient and wanted the heart 'fixed' immediately.

THE ABLATION PROCEDURE

Cardiac ablation is used to treat certain types of arrhythmias. An ablation can be done during open-heart surgery. The more widely accepted method for cardiac ablation uses catheters, long flexible tubes inserted through the groin vein on each leg to travel to the heart to scar or destroy abnormal tissue that produces A-Fib signals. The procedure is done under conscious or general anesthesia and usually lasts five hours.

My ablation was scheduled for November 2nd, 2010 at the University of Iowa Hospital and Clinics. Several things could have kept it from happening. One would have been having a blood clot. A diagnostic test is done to look for clots [PROBABLY A CT ANGIOGRAM). I was to have the diagnostic test right along with blood tests, anesthesia consultation and pre-admission. I would have preferred spending the day with my sister shopping instead of us both in the hospital preparing for a medical procedure. Iodine is injected through the IV into the vein and followed through the body looking for clots.

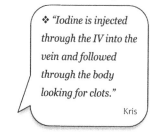

❖ "Iodine is injected through the IV into the vein and followed through the body looking for clots."

Kris

A heart specialist, in addition to the X-ray tech, is present during the procedure for heart patients just in case there are problems. Of course I was having my usual anxiety attack. So the doctor placed a nitroglycerin tablet under my tongue 'just in case'. What an awful taste and horrible headache, but that was nothing compared to the iodine injection. I felt a hot flash go through my body after the iodine was injected into the IV. I felt like I was burning from the inside out, and it lasted longer than I would have liked.

I got very hot in the groin area and was convinced that I had wet my pants. I was expected to hold still the whole time this was happening, though I really wanted a cold shower. I found out how long I could hold my breath when I was told to take a deep breath and hold it until told to breathe normally. I was lying on a table that was moved back and forth through a large noisy rotating circle. The circle was probably three foot wide, so only a portion of my body was in it at a time. What a relief to discover that my jeans were dry when the test was finished. And I didn't have a blood clot, so the ablation could go on as scheduled!

❖ "... 2% to 3% chance...of stroke, death, or other. But those are better odds than living in A-Fib."

Kris

I had to be at the Cardiovascular Clinic at 7 AM the next morning, November 2nd. My sister went with me as my closest relative. She also got custody of my Solara car while I was in the hospital. I think she may have had the better deal – except for the 15 hours she spent waiting at the hospital.

I was having another anxiety attack after being admitted, thinking about what my doctor told me of a 2% to 3% chance of 'something' happening. [SEE EDITOR'S COMMENTS BELOW] He didn't quite define 'something', but I knew it was either a chance of stroke, death, or other. But those are better odds than living in A-Fib. The doctor was cautious and told me that there was a 50% chance that the ablation would be effective. He also thought that I may have to have a second ablation. Fortunately my anesthesiologist gave me a 'happy' med through the IV that the nurse had put in.

Then I met and grilled the Fellow that would be assisting in the procedure. He was a qualified cardiologist, having passed all of the state boards for licensing as well as practiced in the cardiology field. He was studying with my specialist to learn how to perform ablation procedures. He had participated in 20 ablations. His job was to assist the primary physician, my specialist who has over ten years of ablation experience.

IN SINUS RHYTHM!

I remember receiving another dose of meds in my IV along with someone saying it was time to go. That was at 8 AM. The next thing I remember was waking up in recovery. My doctor was standing at the foot of my bed telling me I was in sinus rhythm. But I already knew that the A-Fib was gone by the way my heart felt, the way it beat. I got attuned to the heart rhythm from living with the 'inconvenience' for so long. This was at 4:20 PM. What was considered a five hour procedure actually took over eight hours with prep time and closure.

> ❖ "But I already knew that the A-Fib was gone by the way my heart felt, the way it beat."
> — Kris

I got bits and pieces of the success of the ablation from my doctor, the fellow and the anesthesiologist. My heart went into sinus rhythm of its own accord after the last tissue burns. My blood pressure also crashed when my heart went into sinus rhythm. Sometimes a cardio convert has to be done to get the heart to beat in sinus rhythm after an ablation, but that didn't include me (Yea). My doctor is cautiously optimistic of the success of the procedure. He still maintained that I may need a second ablation down the road for a 'touch up'. He said that a 'flutter' could develop that would need to be taken care of.

> ❖ "He still maintained that I may need a second ablation down the road for a 'touch up'."
> — Kris

RECOVERY

I had a male nurse in recovery whose only task was to take care of me. I had to lay flat on my back so the two 'sites' wouldn't bleed. The site is where the catheter is inserted into the vein. I had two IVs in my arm and an A line (intra-arterial catheter) in my right wrist. The A line is used to monitor blood pressure, take blood samples for testing, and check oxygen saturation. I also had a urinary catheter. I had a vision of my body hooked up to plastic lines, just like in the alien horror movies, during the procedure.

I couldn't comprehend why I had to remind

> ❖ "But my blood pressure had crashed, so I was kept in recovery longer than anticipated."
> — Kris

myself to breath. I had a constant cough. This was from having the breathing tube down my throat. I was given an anti-nausea drug in my IV to help with nausea. I wanted to get up and walk out of the recovery room. There were other patients in the room and one of them would not stop moaning. But my blood pressure had crashed, so I was kept in recovery longer than anticipated.

My family was told that I would be in my room at 5:30 PM but I didn't make it until 7:30 PM. I was confined to lying flat on my back. I wasn't supposed to move for several hours due to the sites' healing process. I wasn't a happy camper being immobile. The nurse did raise the bed a little and then let me elevate my legs around midnight. Good news, I could eat anything that I wanted, as long as it was on the heart healthy menu.

My blood pressure wasn't going up, so I was given fluids to raise it. I wasn't allowed out of bed for some time because my pressure was still low. They were afraid I would pass out. By mid-morning of the next day I finally convinced my nurse to take out the catheter and let me go for a walk. Of course the doctor had to approve it first. The blood pressure dramatically improved after I became the walking water balloon from all the fluid that I was given. It took five days for my legs and ankles to return to normal size. What was scheduled to be an overnight process turned into a three-day marathon because my blood pressure had crashed.

NEW ENERGY AND ATTITUDE—LIVING A "NORMAL" LIFE

I had a dull pain in my heart for the first 24 hours after the ablation. I could have taken a pain killer but I didn't. The pain gradually went away. I did have palpitations the first couple of weeks because I had been in chronic (i.e. Long-standing Persistent) A-Fib. I felt like my heart was attempting to return to A-Fib but couldn't find the electrical pulse to accomplish it.

My sister noticed an immediate positive change in my attitude. I rediscovered the energy that I was accustomed to before A-Fib. The worst outcome from the hospital stay was the sinus infection that I got and my hip/back going out of alignment from lying on a pillow in one position too long. I had developed one heck of a headache that lasted four days.

> ❖ *"I rediscovered the energy that I was accustomed to before A-Fib."*
>
> Kris

I have been taken off all blood pressure meds. I was kept on Coumadin and Prilosec with the addition of Sotalol to slow the heart rhythm. I had to give myself Lovenox shots in the stomach for a week. Lovenox is a blood thinner. I was able to quit taking the Coumadin two months after the ablation and start taking a full aspirin. Hopefully I will be taken off the Sotalol in March [2011]. I am on a very low dosage of Sotalol because it makes me light headed and sleepy. It can make me nauseated. Roughly two weeks after the procedure I woke up with severe stomach cramps which can be an adverse side effect of Sotalol. I do occasionally have stomach cramps which I get to go away by taking a hot shower and staying warm.

I am glad that I had the cardiac ablation. I feel great and have energy to live a 'normal' life. It has lessened the symptoms of my Reynaud's Syndrome, poor circulation in fingers and toes that can cause pallor, numbness, pain and cold extremities.

My quality of life has improved. A friend called me 'bouncy' again, which I had lost during A-Fib. I also know that I need a life style change: no alcohol, watch what I eat, exercise, get plenty of sleep, focus on God and have hobbies to reduce stress among other changes. Life, family and friends are worth the effort!

❖ *"A friend called me 'bouncy' again, which I had lost during A-Fib."*

Kris

Kris
Iowa, USA

Editorial Comments:

Kris' story illustrates the dangers of long-term amiodarone use. When taking amiodarone, make sure your doctor monitors you for possible damage to your thyroid, lungs, liver and eyes. Luckily for Kris, her eye damage was not permanent.

It's normal to be anxious, like Kris, before a Pulmonary Vein Isolation (PVI) procedure. But a PVI procedure is considered low risk, particularly compared to an operation like bypass heart surgery. It has a complication rate of 1%–3% which is comparable to other low-risk procedures such as tubal ligation.

Her doctor was probably a bit conservative in telling Kris she had a 50% chance of being A-Fib free. In most centers the success rate is 70%-85%. If one gets a second ablation, the success rate can go up to 90%. But most people don't need a second ablation.

We're also grateful to Kris for describing how her personal demons of addiction and binge drinking contributed to her Atrial Fibrillation. Her story is both a caution and an inspiration for those fighting both addictions and A-Fib.

A-Fib Returns after 8 years, Opts for Totally Thoracoscopic (TT) Mini-Maze

Daniel thought he had whipped his A-Fib, so after a year he stopped his meds. Eight years later it returned, along with Atrial Flutter this time. Meds were successful, but with unacceptable side effects. He opted for a Totally Thoracoscopic (TT) Mini-Maze operation.

I HAVE HAD Atrial Fibrillation (A-Fib) for 11 years and I have recently gone through a Totally Thoracoscopic (TT) Mini-Maze procedure.[240] I now feel better than I have in years.

I had my first episode of A-Fib in 2000 when I was 48. For the last ten years I had been teaching 7th & 8th grade math and science all day and then I would spend my evenings at school as the technology coordinator. This meant that I would spend hours refurbishing donated computers and running cables all over the campus. These two responsibilities led to a number of 12 hour days. I was also the union president and involved in

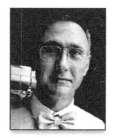

Daniel Doane
Sonora, California, USA

stressful negotiations. My two daughters were teenagers and competitive acrobats; so we often traveled on the weekends to competitions through the state, country, and sometimes internationally.

Needless to say, this was a very stressful time for me emotionally and physically and I was burning the candle at both ends. It all came to a head one Saturday morning when I went running with my wife and realized that my heart was racing at 145 bpm. I could barely stand up. I thought I was having a heart attack. A trip to the emergency room determined that it was Atrial Fibrillation (what the heck is that I thought?) and they were able to convert me using drugs.

I went to my GP who admitted he didn't know much about A-Fib. He sent me to the local cardiologist. He did an echocardiogram and told me I had the healthiest heart he had seen in years and what a pleasure it was to see someone so healthy. He said not to worry about the A-Fib, it wouldn't kill me. He offered no advice for controlling it. By this time I had A-Fib so frequently I was afraid to do anything that was active because it might go off. It would often start in the afternoon and would end when I went to bed.

> ❖ *"I went to my GP who admitted he didn't know much about A-Fib."*
>
> Daniel Doane

Not long after this I had the flu. I awoke one morning and my heart was racing. The A-Fib was very bad, I could barely stand up. I went to the emergency room. The doctor converted me with a diltiazem drip and suggested I talk to my GP about going on diltiazem, a calcium channel blocker. He also said that when you have the flu it can irritate the pericardium, the lining of the heart and make the heart more susceptible to A-Fib. I went on diltiazem and things started improving. Within a few months I was A-Fib free.

I had always been an active guy, but the last few years had been stressful, working a lot of hours, gaining some weight and not being as active. I stopped all caffeine and alcohol because they were obvious triggers for me. I made a concerted effort to simplify my life. I stopped doing all of the tech stuff at school (forcing them to hire someone full time), I stopped all of my union work and all extracurricular school activities. While the diltiazem was controlling the A-Fib, I also noticed that it made me sluggish. And I was gaining more weight. I decided that since the A-Fib had settled down I would lose weight and get in shape. In the next six months I went from 245 lbs. to 200 lbs. and was getting into very good shape. After a year of being A-Fib free I stopped the diltiazem and felt much better. I continued eating well, exercising and not spending any more time at work than necessary.

I really thought I had beat A-Fib. I stayed off coffee and alcohol for years. I would only go into A-Fib if I pushed myself physically for a number of days and got exhausted.

A-FIB RETURNS

In December 2008, when I was 56 years old I stood up from a crouch and went into A-Fib. The next month, the same thing happened in the classroom while I was teaching. I am 6' 2"—so I know when I stand up it takes the blood a little time to catch up with my head and puts a strain on the heart.

Over the next few months I started having A-Fib twice a month, three times a month, then once a week. It would happen when I stood up, when I stretched my arms, or carried my four-year-old grandson on my shoulders.

These were brand new triggers. It got to the point where I would go into A-Fib when I was simply standing still.

> ❖ *"...I began researching A-Fib again. ...I found that there was a specialty, electrophysiology, which dealt specifically with A-Fib."*
>
> Daniel Doane

SERIOUS A-FIB

By August, 2009 I was in serious A-Fib twice a week, 12 hours in bed each time. I had not had much luck with my GP or the local cardiologist, so I began researching A-Fib again.

A lot had changed in the last eight years. I found that there was a specialty, electrophysiology, which dealt specifically with A-Fib. Sacramento is two hours away and has many electrophysiologists. All of the electrophysiologists (EPs) I contacted wanted a referral from a cardiologist, but I didn't want to wait the three months it would take to get in to see the local cardiologist. I found an EP at Sutter Memorial, Dr. Larry Wolff, who would see me without a referral. My appointment was two months away, and my A-Fib was accelerating.

I requested that my GP put me back on diltiazem. It slowed down the A-Fib, but after a month I was an emotional and physical zombie. (It was very deadening. I had no energy and was depressed.) So I had to stop taking diltiazem. This really surprised me because I had taken this same drug for a year at the beginning of my A-Fib and had not had this reaction.

However, that month on diltiazem had broken the cycle, and my A-Fib episodes were now only twice a month and three hours long.

> ❖ *"My EP ... was the first person I talked to who really understood A-Fib."*
>
> Daniel Doane

I made a one page outline of my history and a calendar of each incident of A-Fib and the duration during the preceding year. My EP commented that I had significant A-Fib. He was the first person I talked to who really understood A-Fib. Rather than a specific disorder it seemed to be a spectrum of underlying disorders that expressed themselves in the same way—A-Fib. He said he could manually trigger A-Fib in anyone's heart, but it would stop on its own. The heart substrate would not support A-Fib. My substrate would. The A-Fib wasn't my fault, and I couldn't stop it by avoiding every trigger. "A-FIB BEGETS A-FIB" was the phrase that brought it home to me. Every instance of A-Fib changed my heart, remodeled the substrate, and made it more likely to happen again.

FLECAINIDE AND DIGOXIN WORK

Before I could be considered for a medical procedure, we needed to try a drug approach. I knew my insurance would not approve a procedure until I failed a drug approach. After some testing (echocardiogram and treadmill stress test) my EP started me on flecainide for rhythm and digoxin for rate control. He would have normally used diltiazem for rate, but I couldn't tolerate it based on my most recent experience with it. His next choice would have been a beta-blocker, but I had problems the beta-blocker might worsen. So I ended up with digoxin.

In October, 2009 I started on 0.25 mg of digoxin once a day and 50 mg of flecainide twice a day. This was a starter dose of flecainide to see if I would tolerate it. I started having shorter episodes of A-Fib.

In January, 2010 I went on the full dosage of 100mg of flecainide twice a day and stayed on the digoxin. The A-Fib went away.

DEVELOPS A-FLUTTER

Since I am a school teacher, vacations are when I go crazy with my home improvement projects. I worked like an 18-year-old in the summer heat of 2010, and my A-Fib came back accompanied by a friend, Atrial Flutter. After a week of lugging sacks of ready-mix concrete all over a hillside to set up retaining walls, I thought my A-Fib had come back. But it felt different this time. Normally my A-Fib made my heart feel like a bowl of quivering Jell-O. This time my heartbeat was just very fast, and I was having a hard time catching my breath. My personal rule was that if I went to bed with A-Fib and then woke up with it the next day, I went to the emergency room. That's what I did, and it turned out it was Atrial Flutter.

> ❖ *"This time my heart beat was just very fast, and I was having a hard time catching my breath....it turned out it was Atrial Flutter."*
>
> Daniel Doane

The previous April I had complained to my EP about the digoxin. I was getting headaches, I was tired, and I was getting flashing on the edges of my vision when going from dark to light areas. I asked if I could half my dosage of digoxin. He agreed but he didn't like the idea. He didn't think it would effectively control my rate. I did begin to feel much better, but then the Atrial Flutter hit. My blood tests showed that my level of digoxin had dipped below the therapeutic level. They gave me a shot of digoxin at the emergency room. The nurse just started to push the plunger down when the Atrial Flutter disappeared. Every time I went into one of these bad episodes, I felt like I might not make it. It was very debilitating and scary.

DRUGS WORK, BUT UNWANTED SIDE EFFECTS

I didn't like my medication, but it kept me in NSR which was very important to me. My EP said that even though I had Atrial Flutter, it might have been caused by the flecainide. Sometimes when the heart tries to go into A-Fib, the flecainide can cause it to convert over to Atrial Flutter. He said not to be too concerned about the Atrial Flutter. If it turned out I really had it, he could take care of that with a simple catheter ablation.

> ❖ *"Sometimes when the heart tries to go into A-Fib, the flecainide can cause it to convert over to atrial flutter."*
>
> Daniel Doane

In September 2010, I went on the maximum dosage of flecainide 150 mg twice a day. This was tough. Sometimes I had a very slow heartbeat (35 bpm), skipped beats, was tired, couldn't do mental math and had headaches. While sitting in class I could feel my heart beating very slowly, which it normally did. Then I would start to get a little light headed, and I realized the next beat had not yet happened. I would sit there thinking, "Come on! Beat! Beat!" getting more and more light headed. Then my heart would kick in again, and I would feel better. Other times I would stand up to go to the white board and start to black out. I would have to lean on the white board and just wait. I never did go down, but I was close. Lucky for me I had a great group of kids that year. They never took advantage of my little "quiet times."

I had read that digoxin can cause a decrease in testosterone. So I had my testosterone tested (serum level, never trust saliva testosterone testing). It was low. I started on the usual dose of supplement gel, and it went lower. My urologist finally got it adjusted, and I felt much better. My energy level was up, and the heart meds had caused my A-Fib to settle down. I was A-Fib free from Dec 2010 until late May, 2011.

But I was not happy with the side effects of the drugs as I was now getting daily headaches, and I could tell I was getting more and more emotionally flat. My youngest daughter was getting married at the beginning of the summer. Normally I would have been very excited and enthused about this; but I ended up walking through the preparations, and during the actual wedding I felt like I was one step removed from it all. Every year I produce fifty sets of eight cards of my photographs for my friends and family. When I went to start working on them, I realized I had not taken any pictures all year. However, I still didn't want to switch drugs; because what I had was working for the A-Fib, and I did not want to go into A-Fib again.

DECIDING ON A TT MAZE

Dr. Wolff said he would approve me for a procedure whenever I was ready. My next year was very busy, so I decide to wait for summer vacation. Dr. Wolff recommended that I undergo an operation developed by Dr. Longoria in 2004 at

Sutter Memorial[241] called the TT Maze. Based on what he said and my own research, I agreed. The TT Maze seemed better for my situation rather than a catheter ablation, the TT Maze had a better first time success rate, and the left atrial appendage would be removed, lessening my future stroke risk. I had read time after time about people who were on their second and third failed ablation, and I wanted to try to avoid that.

If my A-Fib had just started, I might have considered a catheter ablation. However, I knew, by the way my A-Fib had returned with such a rapid increase in occurrence and duration and the fact that I would just spontaneously go into it, that the substrate of my heart was prime territory for A-Fib.

Without the medication I think that I would already have moved from paroxysmal to persistent A-Fib. But I could not tolerate the meds any longer. Toward the end of May I began to have short episodes of A-Fib again, so I knew my time was due.

> ❖ *"Without the medication I think that I would already have moved from paroxysmal to persistent A-Fib. But I could not tolerate the meds any longer."*
>
> Daniel Doane

[JUNE, 2011] Dr. Longoria used a model of the heart to show my wife and me how A-Fib occurs. He said that he had done over 180 TT Maze procedures with a 93% cure rate with no A-Fib at all, and those that weren't cured saw great improvement. He talked about other risks, one being the possibility of damage to the phrenic nerve that controls the diaphragm; but that it is unlikely since, unlike a catheter ablation, he can see the nerve. He discussed the fact that I had had an incident of Atrial Flutter; but that this procedure would not cure Atrial Flutter, because that trigger was located inside the right atrium. However, we weren't sure if the Flutter was an artifact of the flecainide. And the Flutter was something that could be dealt with later with a catheter ablation.

The one thing that finally convinced me to go with Dr. Longoria was his patent application (he invented this variation), Methods of Treating a Cardiac Arrhythmia by Thoracoscopic Production of a Cox-Maze III Lesion Set.[242] I found it very useful to read because it describes exactly what may occur. (When asked about the patent, he said he gets no reimbursement from the procedure being used. He applied to limit the ability of companies to market, as their own, the instruments that he helped develop for the procedure; a video of Dr. Longoria performing a TT Maze on OR-Live.com is no longer available but the transcript is very informative.)[243]

BEFORE THE SURGERY

Prior to surgery I needed an echocardiogram, nuclear stress test, lung X-rays, arterial blood sample, meeting with a respiratory therapist and a pint of blood drawn. Dr. Longoria wanted a pint of my own blood in the operating room in the highly unlikely case anything went wrong. I figured, if anything does go wrong, no better person

> ❖ *"Prior to surgery I needed ... a pint of blood drawn. Dr. Longoria wanted a pint of my own blood in the operating room in the highly unlikely case anything went wrong."*
>
> Daniel Doane

to have there than a cardiac surgeon who is working on hearts every day. I also needed a Transesophageal Echocardiogram (which gives a picture of the heart so they can check for clots and clogged arteries), but this would be done just before the surgery when I was under general anesthesia.

THE TT MAZE

July 6, Wednesday 7 AM: I talked with Dr. Longoria and the anesthesiologist. The anesthesiologist said that there would be a branched tube in my throat so they could partly deflate each lung separately. My throat might be a little sore. He was right. It was a bit sore after the surgery, and I was hoarse; but that went away after a couple of days.

They wheeled me into the operating room, and suddenly it was noon. I woke up in recovery. I didn't remember a thing. Dr. Longoria told my wife that at the end of the surgery they were unable to provoke my heart into A-Fib. He said it is no guarantee, but it is a good sign. They transferred me to ICU for one night. I felt better than I normally do when coming out of general anesthesia. The staff was very attentive.

July 7, Thursday: The surgeon's PA [PHYSICIAN'S ASSISTANT] took out the two drain tubes, one on each side of my chest. The drain tubes had not bothered me. I just kept them covered with the sheet and ignored them. I couldn't really feel them. The PA was excellent, no discomfort. Each of the four incisions on both sides of my chest was less than three-fourths of an inch long and tender, but not painful.

They moved me to a room in cardiac recovery. I was up walking by noon. The ICU had started me on the breathing exercises to get my lungs fully inflated, and the nurses kept working with me on that. The most discomfort that I had from the entire procedure was when I would breathe deeply; the left side of the chest was tender. They kept pushing the pain meds so that I could stay ahead of this pain and really work on my breathing. Great advice. As my lungs opened up, I steadily felt much better.

Thursday night was the last night I took a narcotic pain pill. After that I wanted to switch to Motrin, and it worked great.

GOING HOME

July 8 Friday: Dr. Longoria talked with us prior to discharging me. I also had a chance to discuss the surgery with some of the people who had been there. I gathered that I had a number of trigger points all over the right side of my heart that needed to be ablated. They all thought the procedure had gone very well and commented that my heart anatomy was excellent. That had enabled them to see everything very clearly. I didn't need any A-Fib medication, and my heart was steady—no A-Fib. I could go home.

July 9 Saturday: I went grocery shopping and took in a movie with my wife.

ABLATION FOR ATRIAL FLUTTER

Nine days after the procedure I woke up in Atrial Flutter. I had had episodes of Flutter for the last year. Dr. Longoria said that the TT Maze does not ablate the area responsible for Atrial Flutter which is on the inside of the heart. Two days later my EP did

> ❖ "...the TT Maze does not ablate the area responsible for Atrial Flutter...two days later my EP did a right atrium ablation to get rid of the flutter."
>
> Daniel Doane

a right atrium ablation to get rid of the flutter. The procedure was quick and painless. He was probably working on me for only 20 minutes. I was awake during it (on sedation) and was aware of some pressure during the ablation, but had no discomfort or pain. He was optimistic about having gotten rid of the Flutter. I would need to take Multaq and Pradaxa for one month.

RECOVERY

Recovery has gone well. I feel better each day. The emotional flatness from the medications has left me, and my mood is greatly improved. I have energy and my thinking is clear. My heart resting rate had been 42 bpm (this was before I started any meds, I am in good physical condition) before surgery, and now it is 66 bpm. During the TT Maze they needed to ablate nerves coming down the outside of the heart that were playing a large role in my A-Fib. These nerves are also responsible for the release of acetylcholine which helps slow down the heart, so I will never be able to get my rate as slow as it was. I actually prefer the new rate. Previously, I was always aware of my heartbeat. Now it just seems to purr along. It isn't pounding in my chest.

> ❖ *"The A-Fib may return.... I will have catheter ablations done as touch ups for those areas that may reconnect over time."*
>
> Daniel Doane

It has been three weeks since the TT Maze and two weeks since the ablation. I have started interval training on an elliptical and stationary bike. I am starting off slow, capping my heart rate at about 70% max or 115 bpm, but it feels good to know that I can do this. I have been able to get out in the garden and work. I work hard one day and rest the next day. The best part of all of this is that I wake up in the morning feeling happy and optimistic about my day.

Am I cured? Maybe, maybe not. The A-Fib may return, but I feel that TT Maze has done most of the heavy lifting, the Cox-Maze III Lesion-like set that Dr. Longoria uses, along with his own modifications will protect me from A-Fib for quite a while. If and when it does return, then I will have catheter ablations done as touch ups for those areas that may reconnect over time.

WHY DID I CHOOSE THE TT MAZE OVER A CATHETER ABLATION?

If my A-Fib had just started, I would probably have gone with a catheter ablation. After 11 years of A-Fib I was concerned that remodeling had occurred and fibrous tissue had developed. And I wanted the most complete cure I could find.

One EP told me that with catheter ablation it is difficult to make a solid line by burning little points inside a person's heart based on a two dimensional shadow from a fluoroscope. It seems like the incidence of reconnection is much higher for ablations, the procedure can take as much as six to eight hours for complicated cases (they probably worked on me less than two hours). And I think that the skill set required of the EP to be successful is greater than the skill set required of the cardiac surgeon. [SEE EDITOR'S COMMENTS BELOW.]

Plus, my left atrial appendage is gone which reduces my future risk of stroke.

MY ADVICE TO OTHERS WITH A-FIB

There are a few things that I have learned from all of this which I would like to share with others who have Atrial Fibrillation:

Don't blame yourself; you did not make yourself have A-Fib. It is the way your heart is made.

It's the substrate! My EP told me that he can start A-Fib in anyone's heart, but in most people it will just stop. Their hearts won't support it. But ours will. It is fine to avoid triggers and reduce the incidences of A-Fib, but you won't stop A-Fib this way.

Don't believe your GP. I have gotten a lot of bad advice from various GPs:

> ❖ *"Don't believe your GP. I have gotten a lot of bad advice from various GPs:"*
>
> Daniel Doane

    ✗   'Just take a little digoxin and you will be fine.'

    ✗   'You are probably missing some micronutrient. If you buy this product I sell, it may well provide that and stop your A-Fib.'

    ✗   'You need to be on Coumadin if you have A-Fib. Aspirin will not protect you from stroke.' [See editor's comments below.]

    ✗   'I think that all of these tests your EP is requesting are just a waste of money.'

    ✗   (From a cardiologist) 'You have the healthiest heart I have seen in ages. Don't worry about a little A-Fib. It won't kill you.'

If you have Atrial Fibrillation, see an electrophysiologist. If you aren't comfortable with what they are saying, see another one.

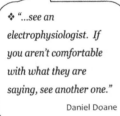

> ❖ *"...see an electrophysiologist. If you aren't comfortable with what they are saying, see another one."*
>
> Daniel Doane

Beware of the hard sell. I once ended up in a hospital that did a lot of catheter ablations, and by the end of my exam I felt like I had been worked over by a car salesman. They could have me scheduled for an ablation in a couple of weeks, and that would take care of all of my problems. In retrospect, I think they were making an effort to increase their numbers and become a high volume center, but their approach made me feel uncomfortable. Fine, I will come back after you are a high volume center.

If you see an EP who does catheter ablations and he/she recommends one and you decide to do it, only go to someone who is the best. Don't let them practice on you. (I got this advice from an EP!)

Don't stay in A-Fib. My rule was if I go to bed with it and wake up with it, I go to the emergency room. If I get it during the day and it is making me dizzy, I go to the emergency room. If it is making me anxious, I go to the emergency room.

If you end up in the emergency room and you have an EP, insist that they call him/her and get a treatment plan. When they come in to take a chest X-ray of your A-Fib, you can say no thanks. My response to them is if my EP wants a chest X-ray, then I will agree to it.

One nurse gave me a smile when I did this and whispered, "It pays to be an informed consumer." Not only is the X-ray unneeded (for my situation), but the radiologist who reads it is not a participating provider for the insurance; so I end up paying extra.

LESSONS LEARNED

I didn't realize how continued A-Fib so drastically remodels your heart. I also didn't appreciate the efficiency and ease of the medical procedures to address A-Fib.

Get your A-Fib taken care of. It won't go away. It may seem to get better, but it will return.

> ❖ *"Get a catheter ablation or a mini-maze procedure, whichever best suits your situation."*
>
> Daniel Doane

Don't think that the medication is a long term solution. Don't put up with nasty side effects. That was the mistake I made. I thought I could tough out the bad part of the medication as long as I stayed out of A-Fib.

Get a catheter ablation or a mini-maze procedure, whichever best suits your situation. I wish I had had this done sooner.

I personally think that the sooner a person has a procedure, the better off they are.

Daniel Doane
Sonora, California, USA

Editorial Comments:

The Totally Thoracoscopic (TT) Mini-Maze is a variation of the Mini-Maze surgery; using four small incisions on each side of the chest, instruments are inserted to make a specific pattern of lesions. But instead of ablating just the Pulmonary Veins as in the Wolf Mini-Maze, lesions and scarring are made in the left atrium to approximate the lesions of the Cox-Maze surgery.

The TT Mini-Maze does not treat Atrial Flutter. To cure Daniel's flutter, a catheter ablation procedure was needed.

Daniel has some good advice about emergency room visits. Keep in mind: on-duty ER doctors may not have the in-depth knowledge and training about A-Fib like your EP. So, talk with your EP and make a plan—under what conditions should you go to the ER, when should you call your EP, etc. While some ER visits may not be needed or advisable (and an unnecessary expense), if there's any doubt, don't stay home and "tough it out." Your peace of mind is important.

If you have A-Fib, you probably need to be on a blood thinner like Coumadin. Aspirin isn't a very effective protection against an A-Fib stroke, but it may be sufficient for people at low risk of an A-Fib stroke.

Like Daniel, you may be comparing the advantages and disadvantages of a Pulmonary Vein Isolation procedure versus a Mini-Maze surgery. In explaining why he chose the TT Maze over a catheter ablation, he made a few arguable comments. Additional information to consider:

- *Difficulty of making PVI point-by-point ablations: Difficult, yes, but electrophysiologists train for this procedure just as surgeons train for making lesions in the Mini-Maze surgery. In addition, during the Pulmonary Vein Isolation procedure, EPs usually verify the integrity of their lesions to make sure there are no gaps. if this is of concern, you may want to consider a CryoBalloon ablation which eliminates the use of point-by-point ablations.*

- *Recurrence rate (return of A-Fib) after a PVI:* Recurrence also occurs with Mini-Maze patients. In fact, some studies indicates a fairly high recurrence rate for Mini-Maze surgeries, i.e., about 35–40% within 6–12 months following surgery. [244, 245] For PVI ablation, studies indicate a 7%–9% chance of A-Fib returning each year out to five years.[246, 247, 248, 249]

- *Procedure time:* Daniels' TT Mini-maze procedure time of 2-hours is indeed notable. While today's Pulmonary Vein Isolation procedures usually take three-four hours, this is a significant advancement—down from four–six hours just a few years ago.

Other considerations when comparing Mini-Maze surgeries and Pulmonary Vein Isolation procedures:

- *Complication risks:* Either choice has the risk of complications. But Mini-Maze surgeries "usually have significant risks compared with catheter-based electrophysiology procedures such as catheter ablation."[250] While the complication rate of catheter ablation is comparable to other routine low-risk procedures[251] such as tubal ligation (1%–2%).

- *Recovery time:* A Mini-Maze is still surgery with significant recovery time first in the hospital and later at home. PVI procedures are less invasive. Some patients go home four-six hours after the procedure, but most go home the next day.

Always consult with your medical advisors before choosing your treatment option.

❖

Two Hematomas + Hemorrhagic Stroke = Worries About Blood Clots

David had a worst case scenario as an A-Fib patient. While on Coumadin, he had a hemorrhagic stroke (bleeding in the brain). He recovered and discovered, like many A-Fib patients, that he could not tolerate blood thinners. But how was he to combat the risk of blood clots and A-Fib stroke without the aid of blood thinners?

IN 2006 WHEN MY heart began to flutter and would not maintain a proper beat, I was referred to Dr. Moussa Mansour at the Cardiac Arrhythmia Center at Massachusetts General Hospital (MGH). There I was diagnosed with A-Fib and began standard A-Fib treatment --- warfarin, aspirin, and, after having my heart shocked back into rhythm (a cardioversion), Sotalol to control my heart rate.

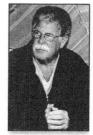

I also had regular INR blood tests monitored by the Anticoagulation Management Services group at MGH to maintain proper levels of blood thinner.

David Berkley
Boston, MA, USA

HEMATOMAS & HEMORRHAGIC STROKE

During the next few years I experienced two hematomas (i.e., a leaking blood vessel), both requiring treatment at the hospital. These hematomas made me fully appreciate the risk of hemorrhaging.

Because of that risk, especially the risk of a stroke, I made it my business to be familiar with the signs of a stroke.

> ❖ *"I made it my business to be familiar with the signs of a stroke."*
>
> David Berkeley

On April 1st 2009 I experienced just such an event, a hemorrhagic stroke (when a blood vessel bursts inside the brain). I immediately called 911. Within 90 minutes of the first symptoms, I was at Massachusetts General Hospital (MGH) where it was determined that the right side of my brain was bleeding.

SOP [STANDARD OPERATING PROCEDURE] relative to this type event was successfully administered. After seven days at MGH and four days at Braintree Rehabilitation Hospital, I was able to go home and continue rehab on an outpatient basis.

Because of my stroke, I couldn't go back on blood thinners like warfarin (Coumadin), but my potential risk of blood clots and A-Fib stroke continued. [TAKING A BLOOD THINNER MAY HAVE CONTRIBUTED TO OR CAUSED HIS HEMORRHAGIC STROKE.]

THE WATCHMAN DEVICE

Currently MGH and Dr. Mansour are participating in an FDA "Investigation" [CLINICAL TRIAL] into the use of the Watchman Left Atrium Appendage Closure Device for A-Fib patients, a device designed to eliminate the need for blood thinners. (MGH and the FDA have info available on line or Google it.)

On April 9th 2010, Dr. Mansour successfully implanted a Watchman LAA Closure Device into my heart. Now, 14 months later, I am pleased to announce that, based on the two Transesophageal Echocardiogram (TEE) tests that have been conducted on my person since that implantation, the "device" is properly placed and functioning as designed.

The Watchman is like a tooth filling. There is no physical sense of its presence. Physically I'm the same. However, now I have some peace of mind.

> ❖ *"Physically I'm the same. However, [with the Watchman] now I have some peace of mind."*
>
> David Berkeley

I continue to take aspirin 325 mg daily and Sotalol but no longer need blood thinners or INR blood testing. I also trust that the risk of a stroke has been diminished. Time will tell.

MY ADVICE

Go to a big city hospital or to a big regional center. I was at the right place, Mass General, and had the right doctors.

David Berkley
Boston's South Shore, MA, USA

Editorial Comments:

For David, drug therapy is serving him well (he has not had an ablation or surgery). Since his cardioversion in 2006, David's A-Fib has been asymptomatic (few or no symptoms). It's still there, but there are no unpleasant effects. He takes aspirin and Sotalol to control his heart rate, and to keep him A-Fib symptom free.

However, the risk of "remodeling" is still there, too. For those on drug therapy for "silent" A-Fib, your heart is still susceptible to electrical and physical changes, and to A-Fib's threat of decreased mental abilities and even dementia (because blood isn't being pumped properly to the brain and other organs). Your heart needs to be checked regularly for enlargement of the atria and for development of Atrial Fibrosis (the formation of fibrous tissue in the heart). Your cognitive abilities should be tracked over time. Remodeling increases your risks of stroke and death, and may require changes to your treatment plan.

After years on standard drug therapy, David had a stroke. There are two main types of strokes: hemorrhagic and ischemic. David had a hemorrhagic stroke, i.e., bleeding in the brain from a burst or ruptured blood vessel. More common is the ischemic stroke caused by a clot in the brain that constricts or blocks off blood supply. Approximately 80%–85% of strokes are ischemic. This is the kind that most often occurs in A-Fib patients.

Blood thinners can cause bleeding in the brain and may have contributed to David's hemorrhagic stroke. But if you have A-Fib and don't take blood thinners, you are five-to-six times more likely to have an ischemic stroke than someone in normal sinus rhythm. A blood thinner like warfarin (Coumadin) reduces the threat of an ischemic stroke by approximately two-thirds.

However, many A-Fib patients needing protection from clots and A-Fib strokes can't tolerate warfarin (Coumadin) or other blood thinners. (In fact, blood thinners are not recommended for 14% to 44% of patients with A-Fib.[252])

If, like David, you can't tolerate blood thinners or just don't want to take them, you do have non-pharmaceutical options. Since most A-Fib clots (90%–95%) originate in your heart's Left Atrial Appendage (LAA), closing off the LAA will reduce your risk of strokes. One option is the expandable Watchman device. It can be permanently implanted, via catheter procedure, at the opening of the LAA to trap blood clots before they exit. This gives about the same protection from an A-Fib stroke as being on blood thinners. For David, it gave him peace of mind, too.

❖

40-Year Battle With A-Fib Includes AV Node Ablation With Pacemaker

Emmett was with the L.A. City Fire Dept. for 27 years. His 40-year story with A-Fib demonstrates, first hand, the recent evolution in the treatment of Atrial Fibrillation including PVIs, AV Node ablation with Pacemaker and, most recently, the Watchman procedure.

I FIRST NOTICED A-FIB in 1972 at the age of 51. At that time I was working 24 hours a day—one day on, one day off. Of course some nights we were up all night. It's quite a strain on the heart to be asleep and suddenly to be out the door on an emergency run in 30 seconds. The A-Fib would often come in spells after heavy exertion. Eventually in 1978, they put me on pension from the Fire Dept. because of the Atrial Fibrillation. However, I did wish very much to continue working at the Fire Department.

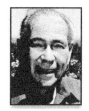

Harry Emmett Finch
Malibu, CA, USA

Many times I had A-Fib at night when I couldn't sleep. I would lie in bed or on the couch. It felt like it would never end. There was almost a feeling of hopelessness. It became so bad that in 1977 I was in three different hospitals and rest homes for a period of almost three months. It is hard to explain, unless a person has it themselves, how difficult and challenging A-Fib can be. It was then that I realized that my heartbeat and breath come only from the creative power we call God, that man himself has very little to do with it other than seek medical help. But medical help, at that time, didn't result in much comfort and alleviation of my A-Fib problem.

> ❖ *"But medical help, at that time, didn't result in much comfort and alleviation of my A-Fib problem."*
>
> Emmett Finch

I was also concerned that A-Fib would occur unexpectedly when I was by myself, or when away from home where the situation could limit or restrict my mobility of movement. There is most often reduced energy and varying feelings of discomfort, as those with A-Fib can testify. This can produce a decided limiting of travel or activities.

During this period my A-Fib was mostly controlled with prescribed meds, good nutrition, and rest if possible. Even so, the episodes would surface occasionally, often daily, with over-exertion or cold drinks. And I found coffee was my enemy. When A-Fib struck, I would try resting, if I could, and take an additional med.

Fortunately, I had watched my diet since my early years, and stayed away from debilitating habits or excesses. My cardiac doctor was well informed, and I trusted in his judgment and expertise to choose what was best for my circumstances. I was always careful in the selection of supplements, hoping for relief, and with proper diet trying to reduce the occasions of A-Fib.

But in my case, the situation worsened as I became older, and the strains of my past careers took their toll. But still, I had faith and belief to make it, with Divine help and hope, along with the medical profession, to aid me.

THREE CATHETER ABLATIONS AND PACEMAKER

My A-Fib worsened; the attacks became more frequent and longer, which of course, caused more concern. Five times in the Spring of 1997, I was taken to the emergency room at St. John's Medical Center in Santa Monica. The A-Fib would go on for as long as 24 hours at a time. I was at the point where I would almost wish to pass on instead of living with my A-Fib.

> ❖ *"I was at the point where I would almost wish to pass on instead of living with my A-Fib."*
>
> Emmett Finch

My cardiologist recommended a new treatment. My first ablation was by Dr. Helmi which helped considerably to reduce the attacks to less than 20 percent of what it was. A Pacemaker was installed at that time. Two and one-half months later, a second ablation was done by Dr. Helmi which kept the A-Fib under control and stopped it for the time being by the use of meds.

But in 2006 I had a bad spell of A-Fib after drinking some coffee, which I usually didn't do. I do believe the coffee triggered the A-Fib, which I had assumed was pretty much cured by the ablation in 1997 and the daily meds.

Then early in 2009, at age 88, the A-Fib re-surfaced and became active again. In March, I had a third ablation at Little Company of Mary Hospital in Torrance, CA, which was unsuccessful. My pacemaker was changed and upgraded hoping to better control the A-Fib, but without much success. In addition, I had two hernia operations in May and July—making it a bit of a strenuous year.

AV NODE ABLATION

By now my A-Fib was becoming much worse, even with prescribed medicines. It is difficult to describe how bad the A-Fib can be, and oftentimes it would last through the night.

> ❖ *"The A-Fib is still with me, only in the background, but not as noticeable or pronounced as before."*
>
> Emmett Finch

I was fortunately referred to Dr. Shephal Doshi in Santa Monica, who did an AV Node Ablation in November, 2009. I felt as if I couldn't have lasted more than a few days without the ablation procedure.

The A-Fib is still with me, only in the background, but not as noticeable or pronounced as before. The A-Fib attacks are not as before, and the heart is paced by the Pacemaker as the result of the AV Node Ablation.

At present the pacemaker is pacing my heart nicely. It's set for 70 and usually doesn't go above 88. But there must be A-Fib or Flutter going on in the background, which tires me out and weakens me to a certain extent. But I don't wish to go through another ablation again.

WATCHMAN PROCEDURE

Later that same year, Dr. Doshi recommended that he insert the Watchman device in my Left Atrial Appendage (that's where the clots are formed).

He's one of the doctors conducting the clinical trial of the Watchman. Because I live by myself, the danger of being cut or injured while on Coumadin (a blood thinner) was of concern to me.

The Watchman device eliminates my need for Coumadin and the chance of a stroke.

> ❖ *"Because I live by myself, the danger of being cut or injured while on Coumadin (a blood thinner) was of concern to me."*
>
> Emmett Finch

LIVING WITH A-FIB

I take Bystolic (a beta blocker) 10 mg morning and evening and Prinivil for high blood pressure. I don't drink coffee, soft drinks, or alcohol. I do take CoQ10, Carnitine, Vitamin E, and Calcium D-3 for bone supplements.

Since the AV Node Ablation and Pacemaker procedure in 2009, my heart feels calm and in rhythm. Two years later at my recent checkup, my pacemaker showed almost no A-Fib episodes at all (I attribute this to my healthy lifestyle including the supplements I take and my faith in a higher power.)

> ❖ *"I am grateful for the technology today that makes this all possible. Otherwise I couldn't be here."*
>
> Emmett Finch

I am grateful for the technology today that makes this all possible. Otherwise I couldn't be here. But through it all, the long experience and battle to overcome A-Fib brought many heart-warming times where I met dedicated, loving and competent members of the medical profession. That, along with the Divine help, sustained me in the dark hours where faith and hope overcame defeat.

LESSONS LEARNED

After dealing with A-Fib for nearly 40 years, I can say that today's modern medicines, along with the different procedures, do much towards lessening the discomfort and limitations of A-Fib. One should not become depressed or without hope for their situation. My faith that a higher power controls the Universe has helped me through the difficulties and challenges of life. This was just another one of those bumps on life's journey. And this one could also be overcome. After all, I had many close calls that nearly terminated my earthly sojourn, from a war (WWII) to the dangers of my firefighting profession.

There is more help available today than when I first developed my A-Fib, and I'm sure more treatment options (like the Watchman device) will be available in the future. Therefore, we should not let fear be our ruler in life.

Harry Emmett Finch
Malibu, CA, USA

Editorial Comments:

Emmett, now an energetic 90-year old, was in his fifties when he developed A-Fib. Over the next forty years he managed his A-Fib and the risk of stroke, first with drug therapy, then with Pulmonary Vein Isolation and AV Node ablation procedures, and most recently with the Watchman device. His story illustrates the quality of life improvements for A-Fib patients through the advancements in the treatment of Atrial Fibrillation.

Though an AV Node Ablation and Pacemaker are generally considered today as a last choice option, it worked for Emmett! The Watchman device doesn't completely eliminate the chance of a stroke, but it does provide much the same protection as being on blood thinners like Coumadin.

Emmett's story is a model for people of faith who look for hope and help from the Divine and use doctors, medicines, supplements, etc. as manifestations of the "creative power we call God."

❖

SUMMARY

Our patients have graciously shared their intimate medical histories with you—their ups and downs along the way, the physical and the emotional tolls, and their progress with this life altering disease. They hope to help you deal with your Atrial Fibrillation, and to help you find your best outcome.

These are just a few of the many personal experiences we have heard over the years—stories of struggle, of courage and perseverance, and of hope—with each patient on their own unique path. For these patients their path led to life improving results.

May these personal experiences strengthen you for the next leg of your journey to finding your A-Fib cure.

In our final chapter, we'll look at the top lessons learned from these A-Fib patients and how to formulate an action plan to find your A-Fib cure.

❖

CHAPTER TWELVE

Your Journey to a Cure

When you study the personal experiences and lessons learned in the previous chapter (and similar stories on A-Fib.com), a consensus of valuable advice emerges. We extracted the numerous gems of wisdom and insight offered up by our A-Fib patients. We grouped the advice by theme, condensed similar thoughts, and trimmed down the number.

What emerged is a consensus—a patients' "Top Ten List" on how to find your A-Fib cure.

A-FIB PATIENTS' ADVICE:
HOW TO FIND YOUR A-FIB CURE

1. Find the best Electrophysiologist (heart rhythm specialist) you can afford.

2. Change doctors if you need to. Don't be afraid to fire your physician.

3. Don't let anyone, *especially your doctor*, tell you that A-Fib isn't that serious, or you should just learn to live with it.

4. Educate yourself. Get the facts about all options before making decisions.

5. Drugs have a role but are not a cure; there are other treatment options that target a cure for your A-Fib.

6. Don't wait—get treatment as soon as possible.

7. Be courageous. Be aggressive.

8. Persevere—try more than one treatment if necessary.

9. Get emotional support to deal with the stress and anxiety, and to help keep up your spirits.

10. Become your own best patient advocate.

So, what do you think of our patients' Top Ten List?

Most of these patients are now enjoying lives free of A-Fib <u>and</u> free of medications. Some of them are content to manage their A-Fib (and risk of stroke) with medication and other techniques. By educating themselves and being their own best patient advocate, these patients found the best outcome for them—they found their "cure."

For many A-Fib patients, their best outcome came about only when they told their doctor, "I want to cure my A-Fib, not just manage it." (And, if needed, they then changed doctors.)

MAPPING YOUR PLAN

You have already begun your journey by reading this book. You now understand the dangers of A-Fib to your health (and to your morale). You're prepared to have an in-depth conversation with your doctor, and to ask the important questions you need answered (and what the answers may mean for you).

You're aware of the various types of meds used to treat A-Fib, their advantages and disadvantages. If you've been prescribed a medication, you now know what kind of a drug it is, how it's supposed to work and its limitations. You know about possible unwanted side effects and what to watch out for.

You know clots and stroke are the immediate danger from A-Fib. (Have you talked with your doctor about your risk of stroke and whether you need to take blood thinners? If not, this should be your top priority. Don't delay on this.)

You've read about all the various treatment options and have probably decided on which options might be best for you. If you're like most people, you probably don't know what caused your A-Fib. But *you do know how to get it fixed!*

> ❖ *Don't let anyone, especially your doctor, tell you that A-Fib isn't that serious, or you should just learn to live with it.*

STEP ONE: TAKE CHARGE

Nobody cares as much as you do about your health.

Don't let anyone, especially your doctor, tell you that A-Fib isn't that serious, or you should just learn to live with it, or to just take your meds. Educate yourself. Learn more about A-Fib and your options.

Know what to ask your doctors. Think about questions in advance of each office visit. Keep a notebook of your questions. Make a list of topics to discuss with your doctor or medical professional. Take your notebook with you to each appointment. Make sure you cover everything on your list. Don't stop until you get your answers. Be a pest, if you must, but get your answers.

Ask about your test results. Learn what the numbers mean, what the target is for a healthy result. Ask for copies of your test reports. Compile them in a file folder or binder for later comparison.

Learn about your healthcare or medical coverage. If necessary, ask your family and friends for help to maneuver through the maze of approvals, referrals, and plan coverage.

As you progress through your treatment plan, continue to educate yourself. Read, surf the internet, participate in online discussions. Become an equal partner with your doctors or health care team.

Remember: Be courageous! Be assertive! Get the care that you deserve. Do NOT go with the flow.

> ❖ *Be assertive! Get the care that you deserve. Do NOT go with the flow.*

STEP TWO: FIND THE RIGHT DOCTOR

Most A-Fib patients should see an Electrophysiologist (EP), a cardiac arrhythmia specialist. An EP is a type of cardiologist focusing on heart rhythm problems —think "electrician" of the heart. (Most cardiologists deal with diseases of the heart and blood vessels—think "plumber" of the heart.) In general, you don't want a plumber fixing your electrical system.

An Electrophysiologist has "more arrows in their quiver" to help you hit your target—a life free of A-Fib. Cardiologists treat arrhythmias with meds (which may not be your best option and shouldn't be your only option). You should think beyond drug therapies. Ideally, you want a life free of A-Fib and free of the threat of heart remodeling—the progressive heart damage associated with A-Fib.

> ❖ *Most A-Fib patients should see an EP (instead of a cardiologist).*

Finding the right Electrophysiologist requires a little work. Not all EPs specialize in Atrial Fibrillation. Some, for example, are pacing interventionalists who work primarily with pacemakers. Others may have their certifications, but do a low volume of catheter ablations for A-Fib and may have limited facilities. Ask your primary care doctors for referrals to EPs, and use the search tools at the Heart Rhythm Society, HealthGrades, Vitals.com or ABMS websites to find specialists near you. (See *Appendix B.*)

However you come up with your list of doctors, you must do your own due diligence. Research each and ask the interview questions for doctors in Chapter Ten.

Note: While many doctors may be equally skilled, not all will find the time to talk with you and answer your questions. If a doctor is too busy to talk with you, in our opinion, they may be too busy to handle your case properly.

It's vitally important that you find a doctor in whom you have confidence, who communicates well with you, someone with whom you can establish an open and honest dialog—someone you can trust.

STEP THREE: AIM FOR A CURE

If you haven't already made a decision, choose which treatment option you want to pursue. Don't postpone for too long. As you already know, A-Fib is a progressive disease that tends to get worse over time. If you let your A-Fib get worse, soon (on the average around a year) it can turn into Long-standing Persistent A-Fib which is harder to fix. Once you make a decision, pursue it as reasonably soon as possible.

> ❖ *A-Fib is a progressive disease. ... Once you make a decision, pursue it as reasonably soon as possible.*

To bolster your resolve, you may want to re-read *Chapter 11: Personal Stories of Hope, Courage and Lessons Learned.* These are the personal experiences of A-Fib patients—people just like you. They have been where you are now. Most are now free of A-Fib (or content with their ultimate choice of treatment).

Consider keeping a diary of your own experience—your path to a life free of the burden of A-Fib.

CONCLUSION

As you already know, as awful as an A-Fib episode may make you feel, normally it isn't going to kill you. And compared to other heart problems, A-Fib is relatively easy to fix.

There are more treatment options than ever before. No longer are you facing a lifetime on medication just putting up with your A-Fib and trying to avoid your triggers. An option such as the Watchman device can help eliminate the need for blood thinners and reduce the risk of stroke.

Catheter ablation procedures offer success rates of 70%–85%, and even higher if you need a second ablation. If you have other heart problems or can't tolerate blood thinners, the Cox-Maze and Mini-Maze surgeries offer equally high success rates. And for A-Fib patients who have tried all other options, an AV Node Ablation with Pacemaker may offer relief from A-Fib symptoms.

But, you need to act. And act soon! A-Fib won't go away on its own. Remember, Atrial Fibrillation increases your risk of stroke.

It's a progressive disease, remodeling and weakening your heart over time, making it harder to cure. Don't let A-Fib rob you of your joy of living. Don't just "take your meds and get used to it."

Armed with what you have learned in this book, you are now empowered to find your cure. You are prepared to ask the right questions, to be persistent until you get the answers, and you're courageous—courageous enough to change doctors if you need to until you find the one right for you.

> ❖ *Many, many former A-Fib patients are enjoying active lives free of the burden of A-Fib.*

You are prepared to be your own best patient advocate!

One final thought: Keep ever in your mind... many, many former A-Fib patients are enjoying active lives free of the burden of A-Fib. You can be A-Fib free, too!

Steve S. Ryan, PhD
Malibu, CA

❖ ❖

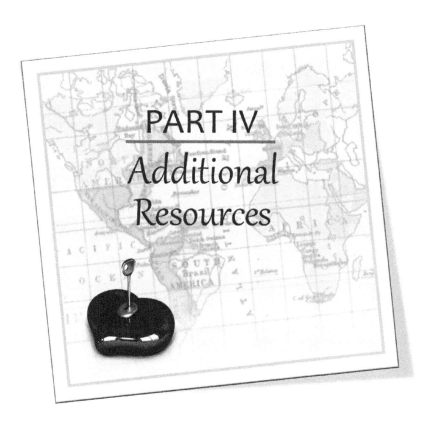

PART IV
Additional Resources

❖

"My recommendation to anyone suffering is
to do your own research, and commence treatment immediately
after finding a qualified physician with a good track record."
Jim, Los Angeles, CA
Free of A-Fib since 2010

❖

APPENDIX A
Glossary of Medical Terms

Ablate:
> To physically destroy tissue or isolate by applications of RF, Cryo, laser, or ultrasound energy.

Ablation:
> A procedure designed to use energy to disrupt or eliminate the faulty electrical pathways that cause abnormal heart rhythms; done through catheters placed into the heart through the blood vessels.

Adrenergic Atrial Fibrillation:
> Atrial fibrillation which usually occurs during the day and is normally triggered by exercise, stress, stimulants, exertion, etc.; related to adrenaline (epinephrine), a hormone and neurotransmitter.

AF or AFib or A-Fib:
> Abbreviations for Atrial Fibrillation.

Anatomically-Based Circumferential Ablation:
> A Pulmonary Vein Isolation strategy; also referred to as Left Atrial Ablation, or the Pappone technique.

Antiarrhythmic Medications:
> Drug therapy that attempts to stop A-Fib and make the heart beat normally.

Anticoagulants:
> Medications such as warfarin (Coumadin) which help prevent blood clots and stroke by slowing the production of blood clotting proteins made in the liver.

Antiplatelets:
> Medications which help prevent blood clots and stroke. An antiplatelet drug works by decreasing the stickiness of circulating platelets (small blood cells that start the normal clotting process), so that they adhere to each other less and are less likely to form blood clots.

Arrhythmia:
> An abnormal heart rhythm.

Arrhythmic:
> Having an abnormal heartbeat; too fast is called Tachycardia; too slow is called Bradycardia; irregular is called Fibrillation.

Arrhythmic drugs:
> Rhythm control drugs used to stop the A-Fib and make your heart beat normally.

Atrial-Esophageal Fistula:

    Abnormal duct or passage in the esophagus wall formed after RF heat damage which is later eroded by gastric acids allowing blood from the heart to leak into the esophagus; a very rare complication (less than one in over 1000 cases) that can be fatal.

Atrial Fibrillation (A-Fib):

    A heart rhythm disorder in which the upper chambers of the heart contract (quiver) very rapidly and irregularly due to chaotic, uncoordinated electrical activity usually originating in the left atrium; a type of supraventricular arrhythmia.

Atrial Fibrosis:

    See Fibrosis.

Atrial Flutter (A-Flutter):

    A heart rhythm disorder in which the upper chambers of the heart (usually originating in the right atrium) contract faster than the lower chambers (the ventricles) in an organized, predictable pattern; a type of supraventricular arrhythmia.

AtriClip from Atritech:

    A surgical device to close off the left atrial appendage (LAA) and reduce the risk of stroke; an alternative to suture or staples.

Atrioventricular (AV) Node:

    Specialized conducting tissue in the right atrium where the atrial and ventricular electrical systems meet; acts as an electrical road or gate connecting the atria to the ventricles; normally the AV Node is the only electrical connection between these heart chambers.

Atrium (plural: Atria):

    Either one of the two upper chambers of the heart in which blood collects before being pumped into the lower chambers (ventricles).

AV Node:

    See Atrioventricular Node.

Beta Blocker:

    A medication that slows down conduction through the heart and makes the AV Node less sensitive to A-Fib impulses.

Blanking Period:

    A two-to-three month recovery period before determining if your ablation was successful.

Blood Thinners:

    Antithrombotic medications which don't actually thin the blood but rather inhibit the ability of substances in blood to form clots.

Bradycardia:

    A heart rhythm problem in which the heart beats slower than normal.

Calcium Channel Blocker:
>A medication that prevents or slows the flow of calcium ions into smooth muscle cells such as the heart; this impedes muscle cell contraction, thereby allowing blood vessels to expand and carry more blood and oxygen to tissues.

Cardiologist:
>A specialist in finding, treating and preventing diseases of the heart and blood vessels; often referred to as the "plumber" of the heart.

Cardiopulmonary Bypass:
>A technique that temporarily takes over the functions of the heart and lungs during surgery, maintaining the circulation of blood and the oxygen content of the body; commonly referred to as a heart-lung bypass.

Cardioversion:
>Converting the heart from A-Fib to normal rhythm by using medications and/or electrical shock.

Catheter:
>A soft, thin, flexible tube about the diameter of a piece of spaghetti (long, thin pasta); For catheter ablations, the tip is equipped with an electrode.

Catheter Ablation:
>A procedure in which a catheter (a soft, thin, flexible tube with an electrode at the end) is inserted through a vein in the groin and moved into the heart; through this electrode, RF or Cryo energy is applied to specific heart tissue to create scars to "ablate" or "isolate" A-Fib signals.

Circumferential Ablation:
>A Pulmonary Vein Isolation strategy in which circular RF ablation lines are made around each pulmonary vein opening to isolate the pulmonary veins and prevent A-Fib pulses from getting into the heart.

Complex Fractionated Atrial Electrograms (CFAEs):
>Low voltage electrical signals with very short cycle lengths used to identify areas in the heart that need to be ablated. CFAEs are increasingly used as targets of catheter ablation; often ablated in addition to and after the ablation of the pulmonary veins.

Cox-Maze Surgery:
>An open-heart operation creating extensive linear incisions on the left and right atria to electrically isolate A-Fib signals to defined paths to the AV Node. Developed by James Cox, MD, in the mid–1980s. Also called "cut and sew maze" or traditional Maze.

Cox-Maze III:
>An open-heart surgery in which the surgeon makes numerous lesions in the atria to isolate A-Fib signals; the current version of the classic Cox-Maze surgery.

Cox-Maze IV:
> The newest refinement of the Cox-Maze; most of the "cut and sew" incisions are replaced with linear ablation lesions created either with radiofrequency energy or cryothermal energy.

Coumadin:
> An anticoagulant; generic name is "warfarin."

Cryoablation:
> An ablation technique that "freezes" the focal sources of A-Fib rather than destroying them with RF energy.

Cryothermal energy:
> A type of "cold" energy used to form lesions or scar tissue in catheter ablation and surgical ablation; works by withdrawal of heat (versus the addition of cold).

Dabigatran:
> A recently FDA-approved drug that acts as an anticoagulant to help prevent clots from forming; does not require close monitoring and has less side effects than warfarin. Expected to replace warfarin as the blood thinner of choice for A-Fib; brand name Pradaxa.

Dallas Extended Lesion Set:
> See Mini-Maze Surgery.

Defibrillator:
> An electrical device that delivers a shock in order to restore the heart to normal rhythm; it is used primarily in life threatening conditions to stop very rapid and irregular heartbeats.

Echocardiography (Cardiac Ultrasound):
> Imaging technology in which special sound waves are bounced off of the structures of the heart; a computer converts them into moving pictures.

ECG:
> See Electrocardiogram.

Ectopic Beats:
> Beats that come from any region of the heart that ordinarily should not produce heartbeat signals (normal heartbeats come from the Sinus Node).

EKG:
> See Electrocardiogram.

Electrical Cardioversion:
> Delivering an electrical shock to the heart in order to convert it from A-Fib to normal rhythm.

Electrocardiogram (ECG or EKG):
> A graphical representation of the electrical activity of the heart. As many as twelve sensors are placed on one's body to record electrical activity from 12 different areas of the heart. An Electrocardiogram is used as an

examination tool to determine if you have A-Fib, and can sometimes show where in your heart an arrhythmia signal is coming from. It is also used during an ablation procedure to determine if an A-Fib signal source has been ablated/isolated.

Electrogram (EGM):

A picture of the electrical activity of the heart as sensed by an ICD or pacemaker implanted in the heart, or produced by catheter mapping devices inside the heart. (This is different from an Electrocardiogram which senses the heart's electrical activity from the surface of the skin.)

Electrophysiologist (EP):

Cardiologist who specializes in the electrical activity of the heart and in the diagnosis and treatment of heart rhythm disorders; the "electrician" of the heart. (Only electrophysiologists with specific training perform catheter ablations.)

Electrophysiology Study (EP or EPS):

A test which uses a catheter inserted through the veins into the heart to determine which areas in the atria give rise to Atrial Fibrillation or Flutter.

Esophageal Fistula:

See Atrial-Esophageal Fistula.

Event Recorder:

A patient-triggered heart monitor/recorder; when feeling an episode of A-Fib, the patient presses a button to record several minutes of the A-Fib episode; also called a loop recorder.

FDA:

See Food and Drug Administration.

Fibrillation:

Rapid, uncoordinated contractions of individual heart muscle fibers.

Fibrosis:

Fiber-like characteristics that develop in place of the normal smooth walls of the heart making you more vulnerable to A-Fib. Not limited to the atria; may occur in the SA node and the AV Node (often leading to Sick Sinus Syndrome).[253]

First-line Therapy:

Based on medical guidelines or protocols, the doctor's typical first choice of treatment.

Five-Box Thoracoscopic Maze:

See Mini-Maze Surgery.

Fluoroscopy:

A special type of X-ray that allows the heart to be visualized on a computer screen.

Flutter:

Rapid, organized contractions of individual heart muscle fibers.

Focal Point Catheter Ablation:
> Early version of Pulmonary Vein Isolation; pioneered in the mid–1990s by Dr. Michel Haïssaguerre of Bordeaux, France.

Food and Drug Administration (FDA):
> U.S. government agency that regulates pharmaceutical drugs and medical devices.

Heart Attack:
> See Myocardial Infarction.

Heart-Lung Machine:
> See Cardiopulmonary Bypass.

Hemmorhagic Stroke:
> See stroke.

Holiday Heart:
> Term used to describe A-Fib and cardiac admissions during or after weekends or holidays when more alcohol is consumed (binge drinking).

Holter Monitor:
> A small, portable heart monitor that records the heart's rhythm continually for 24–72 hours.

Hypertension:
> High blood pressure.

ICD:
> Abbreviation for Implantable (Cardioverter) Defibrillator.

Implantable (Cardioverter) Defibrillator (ICD):
> An implanted electronic device which delivers a shock to the heart any time it senses the heart going into A-Fib; It is also used in patients who have V-Tach (Ventricular Tachycardia).

INR:
> See International Normalized Ratio.

International Normalized Ratio (INR):
> An International Normalized Ratio (INR) is useful in monitoring the impact of anticoagulant ("blood thinning") medicines, such as warfarin (Coumadin); for patients with Atrial Fibrillation, the INR typically should be between 2.0 and 3.0.

Ischemic Stroke:
> See stroke.

Isolation:
> A catheter ablation technique that creates lesions (cuts or scars) around a source of A-Fib to keep it from transmitting A-Fib signals into the rest of the heart. If a source of A-Fib area is "isolated," it is still producing A-Fib signals, but they aren't getting out (spreading) to the rest of the heart.

Lariat II:

>A remote "noose-like" suture delivery system from SentreHeart inserted from outside the heart to close off the Left Atrial Appendage (LAA) and minimize the risk of stroke. It is an alternative to taking blood thinners such as Coumadin (warfarin).

Left Atrial Appendage (LAA):

>A complicated structure located at the top of the Left Atrium and the origin of most A-Fib-related strokes. Blood flow from the Left Atrial Appendage is reduced and impaired by A-Fib leading to the formation of clots which can dislodge and cause stroke.

Lesions:

>In surgery: cuts made with a scalpel (i.e. traditional Cox-Maze); In surgical and catheter ablations: cuts or scars created electronically.

Lone Atrial Fibrillation:

>Describes A-Fib in younger patients (below the age of 60),[254] with no identifiable cause in an otherwise healthy patient; the arrhythmia is the "lone" abnormality present; usually paroxysmal (infrequent) A-Fib.

Long-standing Persistent Atrial Fibrillation:

>When the heart remains in A-Fib continuously for over a year, as contrasted with Paroxysmal A-Fib or Persistent A-Fib (formerly referred to as Permanent or Chronic A-Fib).

Loop Recorder:

>See Event Recorder.

Maze Surgery:

>See Cox-Maze Surgery.

Minimally-Invasive Cox-Maze IV Surgery:

>A variation of the Cox-Maze IV; replaces the "open chest" access (through the breast bone) with small incisions between the ribs.

Mini-Maze Surgery:

>A "keyhole" procedure performed on a beating heart without opening the chest, focused on isolating the pulmonary veins; a modification of the Maze Surgery. Variations include the Wolf Mini-Maze, the Totally Thoracoscopic (TT) Maze, Five-Box Thoracoscopic Maze and the Dallas Extended Lesion Set.

Myocardial Infarction:

>A total blockage of blood flow and oxygen to a portion of the heart which damages the heart's muscle cells.

Normal Heart Rhythm:

>See Normal Sinus Rhythm.

Normal Sinus Rhythm (NSR):

>The normal beating of the heart (60–100 beats per minute); also called Sinus Rhythm.

NSR:
> See Normal Sinus Rhythm.

Operating Room (O.R.) Report:
> A very technical, detailed report by your electrophysiologist or surgeon which describes step-by-step the results of a particular procedure or surgery. (Because it is very technical and difficult for patients to read, it isn't normally given to patients unless they ask for it.)

Ostium (plural Ostia):
> The opening from a pulmonary vein into the left atrium.

Pacemaker:
> A small, implantable device that provides an electrical stimulus to the heart when the natural electrical signal is absent or too slow to provide sufficient pumping action.

PACs:
> See Premature Beats.

Paroxysmal Atrial Fibrillation:
> Occasional attacks of A-Fib that return to normal heartbeat (sinus rhythm) on their own (as contrasted with Persistent A-Fib or Long-standing Persistent A-Fib).

Pericarditis:
> Inflammation of the sac that surrounds the heart (the pericardium).

Permanent Atrial Fibrillation:
> Often refers to patients where a decision has been made not to pursue restoring the heart to normal rhythm by any means including catheter or surgical ablation.

Persistent Atrial Fibrillation:
> A-Fib that lasts for over a week, or A-Fib that lasts less than a week and requires cardioversion to return to normal sinus rhythm.

Pill-in-the-Pocket:
> Drug therapy in which the patient takes an antiarrhythmic med at the time of an A-Fib attack; a variation of the Pill-in-the-Pocket treatment is to take an antiarrhythmic med on a regular basis, then take a higher dose at the time of an A-Fib attack.

Polar Heart Rate Monitor:
> A consumer device for monitoring one's pulse rate. Designed primarily for runners, it consists of a band worn around the chest which transmits a signal to a special wrist watch. The watch can be set to sound an alarm if the runner's pulse rate goes too high. Has been used by patients to detect their A-Fib episodes. Available in sporting goods stores.

Post-Operative A-Fib:
> Atrial fibrillation which arises during or soon after cardiac surgery; generally, it stops by itself, but sometimes the patient may require treatment.

Premature Atrial Contractions (PACs):
>See Premature Beats.

Premature (Extra) Beats:
>Premature beats that occur in the atria (the heart's upper chambers) are called premature atrial contractions, or PACs. Premature beats that occur in the ventricles (the heart's lower chambers) are called premature ventricular contractions, or PVCs. In a normal, healthy heart premature beats happen naturally and are considered benign. However, some heart diseases can cause them. They also can be caused by stress, caffeine, nicotine, or too much exercise.

Premature Ventricle Contractions (PVCs):
>See Premature Beats.

Pulmonary Vein:
>One of four veins that brings oxygenated blood from the lungs into the left atrium. (The openings from these Pulmonary Veins into the left atrium are the source of most A-Fib signals).

Pulmonary Vein Antrum Isolation (PVAI):
>A Pulmonary Vein Isolation strategy in which the pulmonary vein openings are ablated in pairs with very wide lesions in the Antrum rather than near the vein openings.

Pulmonary Vein Isolation (PVI):
>Catheter ablation procedure to isolate A-Fib signals by abating the openings around the pulmonary veins; also called Pulmonary Vein Ablation (PVA).

Pulmonary Vein (PV) Potentials:
>An electrical charge or energy (potential) in the Pulmonary Vein openings that can cause A-Fib. PV Potentials can be measured and pinpointed even if the patient isn't in A-Fib at the time.

Pulse Oximeter:
>A medical device that monitors the oxygen saturation of a patient's blood. Most monitors also display the heart rate.

PVCs:
>See Premature Beats.

PV Stenosis:
>Swelling of the Pulmonary Vein opening that may occur after catheter ablation. This swelling is permanent and can restrict blood flow from the lungs into the heart.

Radio Frequency (RF):
>High frequency electrical energy used to form lesions or scar tissue in catheter and surgical ablations.

Rate Control Medications:
>Drug therapy that attempts to control your heart rate (ventricular beats), but may leave the upper chambers (atria) of your heart in A-Fib.

Recent-Onset Atrial Fibrillation:
> Term used to describe A-Fib during the first 48–72 hours of occurrence.

Recurrence:
> Return of symptoms of a disease.

Remodeling:
> Electrical, contraction, and structural changes to the heart, including enlargement of the atria and development of Atrial Fibrosis.

Rhythm Control Medications:
> Drug therapy that uses rhythm control drugs, called antiarrhythmics, to try to stop the A-Fib and make the heart beat normally.

Segmental Catheter Ablation:
> A Pulmonary Vein Isolation strategy that uses Pulmonary Vein Potentials to identify and ablate (destroy) focal points or areas of the heart producing A-Fib signals.

Septum:
> A thin membrane separating the right and left atria; during a PVI procedure, the septum wall is pierced to allow the catheter to advance from the right atrium into the left atrium.

Silent A-Fib:
> Atrial Fibrillation in which the patient feels no or very few symptoms; often discovered only during a routine medical exam.

Sinoatrial (SA) Node:
> See Sinus Node.

Sinus Node:
> A specialized group of cells in the heart which generates an electrical signal that travels down a single electrical road (the AV Node) connecting the atria to the ventricles. The Sinus Node is called the heart's "natural pacemaker," because it maintains a regular heartbeat and makes adjustments to increase the heart rate during exercise and to slow it during rest. Also called "Sinoatrial (SA) Node."

Sinus Rhythm:
> The normal beating of the heart (60–100 beats per minute); Also called "Normal Sinus Rhythm," (NSR).

Stenosis:
> A swelling, constriction or narrowing of a duct or passage. See PV Stenosis.

Stroke:
> There are two main types of strokes: hemorrhagic and ischemic. Hemorrhagic stroke is caused by a leaking or ruptured blood vessel in the brain. More common is the ischemic stroke caused by a clot in the brain that constricts or blocks off blood supply. A-Fib related strokes are most often Ischemic.

Structural Heart Disease:
> One of several different structural defects in the heart including heart muscle disease (cardiomyopathy), heart valve disease, congenital heart disease (patients born with abnormalities of the heart valves or chambers), and heart damage caused by infection, such as Pericarditis.

Symptomatic Atrial Fibrillation:
> Atrial Fibrillation with noticeable symptoms (versus asymptomatic or Silent A-Fib).

Tachycardia:
> A heart rhythm problem in which the heart beats faster than normal.

TEE:
> See Transesophageal Echocardiogram.

TIA:
> Transient Ischemic Attack, a temporary "mini-stroke."

Totally Thoracoscopic Maze:
> See Mini-Maze Surgery.

Transesophageal Echocardiogram (TEE):
> Test for the presence of blood clots in the heart; a tube is run down the esophagus next to the heart; the echocardiogram uses high-frequency ultrasonic waves from within the esophagus to visualize structural and functional abnormalities of the heart.

Transmural Lesion:
> Lesion or scar that passes through or completely penetrates the entire thickness of the atrial wall (heart tissue).

Ultrasound:
> High-frequency sound vibrations used in some imaging technologies and catheter-based procedures.

Vagal Atrial Fibrillation:
> A form of A-Fib that occurs at night, after a meal, when resting after exercising, or when you have digestive problems; related to the Vagal nerve.

Ventricles:
> The two lower chambers of the heart.

Ventricular Tachycardia:
> A fast heart rhythm that originates in one of the ventricles. It is a potentially life-threatening arrhythmia, because it may lead to Ventricular Fibrillation—very rapid uncoordinated fluttering contractions of the ventricles resulting in loss of synchronization between heartbeat and pulse beat. Unlike A-Fib, it can be very dangerous and result in sudden death.

Warfarin:
> The generic name of the anticoagulant "Coumadin."

Watchman:
> A device from Atritech inserted via catheter which closes off the Left Atrial Appendage to minimize the risk of stroke. It is an alternative to taking blood thinners such as Coumadin (warfarin).

Wolf Mini-Maze Surgery:
> A version of the Mini-Maze surgery developed by Randall Wolf, MD; see Mini-Maze Surgery.

APPENDIX B

Recommended Resources
& Website Links

We personally reviewed hundreds of resources and websites before selecting these to complement the information in this book. These recommendations offer you additional resources that go beyond the margins of this manuscript.

In addition to informational and research websites, you'll find animations, audio clips and short videos, online tools, services and networking opportunities.

Note: The URL web address for each online resource is listed in the Bibliography under Online Resources.

Our recommendations are divided into categories and listed in alphabetical order.

- Discussion Groups, Forums, and Message Boards
- Information Services
- Informational Websites
- Instructional Audio and Video Clips
- Online Tools
- Reference Books and Reports

Caution: when surfing the net, recognize that some sponsors of A-Fib-related websites may be biased toward a particular technique, pharmaceutical, or medical device (often for financial gain). Always ask yourself, "Who is paying for this website? And what is their agenda?"

DISCUSSION GROUPS, FORUMS, AND MESSAGE BOARDS

A-Fibcures–Non-Pharmaceutical Cures for A-Fib: a forum on Yahoo! with emphasis on the Cox-Maze and Mini-Maze Surgeries.

AFIBsupport: a support group on Yahoo! for patients and others interested in A-Fib. It includes useful databases and information.

Lone Atrial Fibrillation Bulletin Board: is dedicated to Lone A-Fib but covers many subjects relevant to anyone with A-Fib; from The AFIB Report.

The Heart Forum: for questions and support regarding heart issues, including A-Fib. Questions are answered by doctors from the Cleveland Clinic.

INFORMATION SERVICES

CenterWatch: global source for clinical trials information for professionals and patients.

ClinicalTrials.gov: listing federally funded and privately supported clinical trials; a service of the National Institutes of Health (NIH).

Google Scholar Alerts: select keywords or phrases and Google Scholar automatically emails you links to new material (independent of publication date) that has just "entered" the database. (Keywords such as Atrial Fibrillation, CryoBalloon ablation, Cox-Maze IV, etc.)

MyConsult Online Medical Second Opinion: fee-based service (around $600.00) from the Cleveland Clinic (Not available in all US states, nor internationally).

INFORMATIONAL WEBSITES

AFAnswers: includes diagnosis and treatment information; by St. Jude Medical.

Arrhythmia Alliance (UK): well written general info on heart arrhythmias and A-Fib.

Atrial Fibrillation Association–US: branch of the UK non-profit organization; general patient and clinician information on established, new or innovative treatments for A-Fib.

Atrial Fibrillation–Resources for Patients: the author's website; array of information for patients with A-Fib; includes extensive list of Electrophysiologists/Facilities sorted by U.S. states and internationally; by Steve S. Ryan.

Choosing a Non-Drug Treatment for Atrial Fibrillation: good analysis of catheter ablation and surgical options to cure A-Fib from AF-Ideas.com by Dick Inglis.

Cleveland Clinic Center for Atrial Fibrillation: review of A-Fib basics.

Heart Care Centers of Illinois: very clear explanation of A-Fib and the Pulmonary vein Isolation procedure.

> **CAUTION**
> ❖ Some A-Fib-related resources may be biased toward a particular technique, pharmaceutical, or medical device (often for financial gain). Always ask yourself, "Who is paying for this website? And what is their agenda?"

Heart Rhythm Society: Includes educational section for patients with A-Fib, and a "Find a Specialist" search tool.

London Atrial Fibrillation Centre: good explanations and graphics of A-Fib (where former British Prime Minister, Tony Blair, was treated for his arrhythmia).

MedlinePlus/Arrhythmia: accumulates information on A-Fib from the National Library of Medicine (NLM), the National Institutes of Health (NIH), and other U.S. government agencies and health-related organizations.

Medscape Today: excellent articles, research, and expert medical opinions on A-Fib (free membership required).

The American Heart Association: Arrhythmia/heart disease information.

Your Rights To Your Medical Records Under HIPAA: Fact Sheet (for U.S. residents).

INSTRUCTIONAL AUDIOS AND VIDEOS

Atrial Fibrillation Patients Who Do Not Respond to Antiarrhythmic Drugs Should Be Treated with Catheter Ablation: three-minute video clip from Insidermedicine.

Atrial Fibrillation: excellent one-minute animation of the normal heart and the heart in A-Fib; by CardioChoices Channel/Boston Scientific.

CryoAblation Balloon Catheter: video dramatization of the balloon catheter in use; from Medtronics.

How the Healthy Heart Works: excellent one-minute animation of how the healthy heart works; from St. Jude Medical Health.

Listen to a Heart: Sound of the heart in A-Fib (head set recommended) a .wav file from Case Western Reserve University; Compare to *Normal Heart Sounds* from Asada Sensei on YouTube.

Overview of Atrial Fibrillation: nine minute instructional video about Atrial Fibrillation; good animation of the normal heart and the heart in Atrial Fibrillation; from wired.MD®.

Pulmonary vein Isolation Procedure: 5:30 min. video about a patient's PVI procedure; from UCLA Cardiac Arrhythmia Center.

Stepwise Approach to Interpreting an ECG: excellent six-minute video shows how to interpret an ECG; from Insidermedicine.

Your Heart's Electrical System: two-minute video animation identifies the parts of the heart and illustrates the role of each, and shows how clots form; from the National Heart Lung and Blood Institute.

ONLINE TOOLS

ABMS Certification Matters: specialist locator and research online tool for Electrophysiologists; verify a doctor's Board Certification; by American Board of Medical Specialists; Toll-free service 866–ASK–ABMS (866- 275–2267).

DoYourProxy.org: free online generator tool for health care proxy document; create a fully-customized document.

Google Scholar: provides a simple way to broadly search for scholarly literature, i.e., medical journal articles, scholarly papers, and scientific research studies and presentations;

HealthGrades: an independent healthcare ratings organization provides physician's profile, education, patient reviews, awards & recognition, insurance accepted, hospital affiliations, malpractice or sanctions, locations.

HRS Finding a Doctor: specialist locator tool (U.S., Canada, or International) by the Heart Rhythm Society.

Medical Alert I.D. Wallet Card: free online generator tool for fully customized medical info wallet card.

PubMed/Medline.gov: a biomedical literature search engine from U.S. National Library of Medicine National Institutes of Health.

Vitals.com: specialist locator and research online tool; options to search by gender, language spoken, or insurance provider; by MDx Medical, Inc.

REFERENCE BOOKS AND REPORTS

Atrial Fibrillation: The Latest Management Strategies, Hugh G. Calkins, M.D. and Ronald Berger, M.D., Ph.D. Special Report from Johns Hopkins, (University Health Publishing–MediZine, NY, NY.) 2011. Digital PDF document.

The Patient's Guide to Heart Rhythm Problems, Todd J. Cohen, Johns Hopkins University Press, 2010.

MediFocus Guidebook on Atrial Fibrillation, Elliot Jacob (Editor). Medifocus.com, Inc. 2011. Kindle Edition.

❖

Note: online destinations and content change without warning. Websites and web addresses are current as of our publication date.

❖

APPENDIX C

Finding My A-Fib Cure
by Steve S. Ryan

Steve Ryan had his first A-Fib attack in early 1997. He was 56 years old and was in apparent good health (5'10", 185 lbs.). He trained for and ran 400 meter dashes and 5K's. He and his wife resided in Los Angeles, California. He worked on the camera crew of the NBC soap opera "Days of Our Lives" which involved frequent late nights and overtime. Cured of A-Fib in April, 1998, this is his story in his own words.

THE FIRST TIME I HAD a noticeable attack of A-Fib was Sunday evening January 19, 1997. It felt like I had mice running around in my heart. My pulse would get weird and irregular, then start racing. Just days earlier I had undergone laser surgery on my face and was in a lot of pain. I can't think of anything else that might have triggered the A-Fib.

Steve S. Ryan, the author

JANUARY 1997

By the time I got to a hospital emergency room that Sunday evening, my pulse was nearly back to normal and I was sent home. My physician, Dr. Glenn Gorlitski, sent me to a specialist, Dr. Robert Levin with Cardiology Consultants of Santa Monica. On Friday, January 24, as soon as they hooked me up for a treadmill test, they could see from the ECG that I had A-Fib.

MY DIAGNOSIS

I had "Paroxysmal" A-Fib (episodes that stop on their own, and last anywhere from seconds or minutes, to hours or up to a week). My A-Fib attacks would usually be short but would recur frequently, sometimes around twenty a day. Other days I wouldn't have any attacks. Every once in a while I'd feel lightheaded and almost lose consciousness. I later found out that, after an episode of A-Fib, my heart would sometimes stop beating for several seconds before kicking into normal rhythm.

Dr. Levin prescribed the blood thinner warfarin (Coumadin 5 mg) for me to make sure I didn't have a stroke. (In A-Fib, the chambers of your heart aren't pumping out properly. Blood clots can form and travel to your brain causing a stroke. Blood thinners like Coumadin and aspirin help keep these clots from forming.)

> ❖ *I was on and off several different medications. None of them seemed to do much good.*

During this time I was on and off several different medications. None of them seemed to do much good.

They were:

1. Toprol-XL (metoprolol) 50 mg (a class II beta-blocker)
2. Digoxin (Lanoxin 0.125 mg)
3. Quinidine Glaconate (quinidine) 324 mg (class 1A)

4.   Procanbid (procainamide) 1000 mg (class 1A)
5.   Betapace (sotalol) 80 mg (a class II and class III drug)
6.   Cordarone (amiodarone) 5 mg (a class III and class I drug)

Toprol-XL did slow down my heart rate significantly. My pulse got down in the 30–40 beats per minute range which isn't healthy. I still had A-Fib but it slowed down along with my pulse. Cordarone (amiodarone) made me impotent and caused me to cough up blood.

OCTOBER 1997: DISABILITY LEAVE

Since I worked around heavy, moving equipment, I had to stop working and go on disability. This really motivated me to find a cure.

At this point my life was pretty much in the tank. In addition to having to quit work, I had to give up training for the 400 meter dash and all sprinting. I still tried to jog while wearing a heart monitor (Polar Heart Rate Monitor available in sporting goods stores). If I went into A-Fib when I started jogging, I'd stop and just walk for a while. When I'd go into A-Fib, I'd first feel a fluttering sensation in my chest; then shortly afterwards my pulse would jump from 60 to 120 or higher. Being dedicated to running I'd sometimes run with A-Fib. My pulse would be very fast during the whole run. This probably wasn't a smart thing to do. A lot of time when relaxing after a run, I'd go into A-Fib.

NOVEMBER/DECEMBER 1997: TWO FAILED AND ONE ABORTED ABLATION

Dr. Levin sent me to Dr. Ibrahim Helmy, an Electrophysiologist at St. John's hospital in Santa Monica. He performed catheter ablation procedures on me on two occasions, November 18 and December 8, 1997. He only worked in my right atrium to eliminate Atrial Flutter (which I wasn't diagnosed with). These procedures seemed unsuccessful to me. (It wasn't until later that I learned ablations in the right atrium have very little chance of curing A-Fib, which generally originates in the left atrium. "Waste of time" comes to mind, but to be fair, this was 1997, early in the development of the procedure).

He referred me to Dr. Wee Nademanee at the USC Medical Center who tried to perform a catheter procedure on December 16, 1997. He attempted to get into my left atrium but had equipment problems (his hard drive crashed forcing him to stop; but I think the EP was also having difficulty getting a catheter into my left atrium). [SEE EDITOR'S COMMENTS BELOW]

MY RESEARCH BEGINS WITH A VENGEANCE

Now I was discouraged and even desperate. My wife, Patti, encouraged me to get on the Internet and research Atrial Fibrillation for myself, instead of relying on my medical advisors. I did this with a vengeance. Armed with a medical dictionary, I spent a lot of time in medical libraries reading everything I could find about A-Fib including medical journals, medical text books, and medical research papers. I even learned to read my own ECG.

> ❖ Now I was discouraged and even desperate.

I copied all my medical files and sent them to every US doctor and researcher in A-Fib who might help me or give me information. I spoke with each over the phone.

Ultimately, I consulted and was examined by additional doctors including Dr. Christopher Wyndham of the North Texas Heart Center in Dallas, Texas; Dr. Richard Page at the University of Texas Southwestern in Dallas, Texas; and Dr. Tony Pacifico at Baylor University Medical Center in Houston, Texas.

MARCH 1998: SEARCH LEADS TO BORDEAUX, FRANCE

My research and conversations with experts in A-Fib eventually led me to look for my cure outside the U.S. The world leader in the treatment of A-Fib was in Bordeaux, France, Dr. Michel Haïssaguerre. (The very first article I read and doctor I talked to, Dr. Frank Marcus of the University of Arizona, mentioned Dr. Haïssaguerre's work. But at that time it never occurred to me to contact Dr. Haïssaguerre directly. Going to Bordeaux, France, for treatment seemed like going to Mars!)

> ***** NOTE**
> During this timeframe (1997-1998), *Focal Point Catheter Ablation* wasn't an FDA-approved procedure in the United States (but was being performed in FDA clinical trials). ❖

After months of research and talking to other doctors, I finally decided to see if Dr. Haïssaguerre could help me.

Writing and faxing to a hospital in Bordeaux, France, wasn't all that difficult, but calling on the phone was quite a challenge even though I thought I knew enough French. After reviewing my records, ECGs, etc., Dr. Haïssaguerre thought I would be a good candidate for a Focal Point Catheter Ablation* procedure (early version of Pulmonary Vein Isolation/Ablation).

In his research and practice he had identified areas of the heart that produce the extra pulses of A-Fib. He would pass a catheter from the groin up through a vein to the heart, then using RF energy he would cauterize or isolate the diseased heart tissue that was producing the extra pulses. He had a good deal of experience with this procedure.

It was quite a mental leap for me and my wife to even consider going outside the U.S. for treatment. We had to find out how much it would cost, and whether my insurance would cover any or all of it. I was very fortunate to be covered through my company GE/NBC by Blue Cross/Blue Shield of Alabama. Once they got all the information they needed, I was pre-approved for treatment in France, though of course we had to pay for travel and lodging. (The final bill in 1998 for twelve days including two major and two minor procedures in the Bordeaux hospital was $9,235.04, far less than we would have paid in the U.S. We paid the bill by credit card. My GE/NBC insurance later reimbursed me 100%, though I first had to translate the bill from French to English.)

> ❖ *It was quite a mental leap for me and my wife to even consider going outside the U.S. for treatment.*

A cancellation in their schedule opened a slot for me sooner than expected. Imagine—we had to get updated passports, make travel and lodging arrangements, work out how to pay the French hospital, etc. in just a few weeks. The biggest obstacle came from a company called United Health Care which administers GE/NBC's disability program. Because A-Fib frequently reoccurs after the first procedure, Dr. Haïssaguerre requested I stay in the hospital in France for eight–ten days (I actually wound up staying longer). But United

HealthCare insisted on a return to work date earlier than that. I could have lost my job if I was absent without leave. But thanks to the Family Medical Leave Act and a sympathetic manager at GE/NBC, I was able to get an unpaid leave of absence from work and later return to my same job.

APRIL 1998: FRANCE HERE WE COME

My wife, Patti, and I flew into Paris Friday, April 16, then took a train (the TGV) to Bordeaux. I was due to check into the French hospital Sunday, April 19, but I showed up there Saturday to make sure we could find our way and get to the right department. When I checked into L'Hôpital Cardiologie de Haut-Lévèque, Ave. de Magellan, 33604 Bordeaux-Pessac on Sunday, my A-Fib symptoms had disappeared! (While few Bordeaux residents spoke English, Dr. Haïssaguerre did.) He reassured me that this was not unusual, that 30% of his patients have the problem of disappearing symptoms when they arrive.

Hôpitaux de Bordeaux

Everyone at the hospital was remarkably friendly, though very few spoke English. They gave me a big room with two beds so that my wife, Patti, could stay with me when she wanted. The food was incredibly good. Almost every dish had its special French sauce. Someone arranged that I get double portions of the entrees which I very much appreciated. The nurses' stations seemed well staffed with competent, caring nurses.

TESTING BEGINS

On Monday and Tuesday I went through several tests and monitoring procedures in preparation for my catheter ablation procedure which was scheduled for Wednesday. They took X-rays and set me up with an RF heart monitor that allowed me to stroll around rather than be confined to bed. I took advantage of this to explore the hospital grounds which were very scenic. (One time when I walked into an elevator, the floor nurses ran around looking for me because they had lost the RF signal. From then on I told the

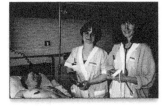

Two of my nurses and me in Bordeaux, France

floor nurse any time I was going to use the elevator.) I also had a 12–lead battery-operated ECG on for a day. Sometimes I also had on a Holter monitor which records your heartbeats when you press a button. I had so many monitor electrodes on my chest you could hardly see the skin. But I still wasn't experiencing any A-Fib symptoms. They had me do ten squats with the ECG leads attached, but even that didn't work.

My lead doctor, Dr. Michele Haïssaguerre

Everyone warned me about the test I'd have to take on Tuesday. I would have to swallow an Ultrasound (Doppler) tube which would be used to check for blood clots in my heart. If any were found, they couldn't do the procedure. I gargled an anesthetic, then I had to swallow this huge tube. It was tough not to gag on it. After what seemed like an awfully long time, they finally pulled out this tube and told me they found no blood clots in my heart. Even the stress of this test didn't bring on any A-Fib attacks. Later that day they put me on a stationary bike, but I still wouldn't go into A-Fib.

Dr. Haïssaguerre reassured me that he had other means of stimulating my A-Fib, and that this was one of the reasons he had asked me to plan on staying eight–ten days in the hospital. He also told me I would be awake during the entire catheter ablation procedure so that I could interact with the doctors, give feedback, etc. Tuesday evening a nurse came in and shaved off every hair around my groin.

PROCEDURE DAY ARRIVES

Wednesday morning, April 22, my catheter ablation procedure began. In my room the attendant put me on a gurney and wheeled me into the elevator and down to the procedure room, then he and a nurse transferred me to the operating table. The nurses made me as comfortable as possible, since I might be on my back for a long time. One nurse wore a lead shield, and they all worked behind some kind of glass or plastic shields. I wondered how much fluoroscopy radiation I would be exposed to as they used the fluoroscopy to guide the catheter through my heart.

They gave me a local anesthetic in my groin and made a small cut in a vein there and inserted the catheter. I was relieved that it didn't hurt much at all. Dr. Haïssaguerre tried to induce me into A-Fib, first with a hormone similar to that produced during exercise, then with a drug that made me feel somewhat dizzy and strange. On his cue I pushed and held my breath. But nothing worked.

Finally, using the catheter he stimulated me into A-Fib. But once started, the A-Fib wouldn't stop. After 20 or 40 minutes and use of an intravenous medication, the A-Fib stopped. Shortly thereafter I spontaneously went back into A-Fib which is exactly what they wanted. The heart tissue that was producing these extra pulses was identified as the right superior pulmonary vein ostium area (an opening from one of the veins coming from the lungs into the heart).

Anytime something changed or when they started a new procedure, Dr. Haïssaguerre or his colleague, Dr. Shah, would walk over and talk to me about what they were doing, what I should expect, what I might have to do, and to ask me how I was doing. Their care and attitude was incredibly reassuring and made me feel confident. I had certainly come to the right place. (They spoke among themselves in a combination of French, English, and what I think was a Bordeaux dialect that was unrecognizable to me. Sometimes, like when I went into spontaneous A-Fib, it sounded like a French soccer match with all the cheering! They certainly had a great camaraderie and enthusiasm for what they were doing.)

❖ *Their care and attitude was incredibly reassuring and made me feel confident. I had certainly come to the right place.*

Dr. Pierre Jaïs, a colleague of Dr. Haïssaguerre, guided the catheter from my right atrium through the transseptal wall (the heart tissue that separates the right and left atrium) and into my left atrium in less than five minutes. This is a rather tricky procedure in which he was obviously very skilled and experienced. Then Dr. Haïssaguerre took over. With RF energy from the catheter tip, he cauterized part of the area of my right superior pulmonary vein ostium. He told me that the tissue there did look diseased. He also checked all the other typical focal point areas of the heart, but they looked OK. They gave me some medication so that I wouldn't feel the burning in my heart tissue.

With someone who is continuously in A-Fib, they treat the tissue and the A-Fib stops— indicating the diseased tissue has been cured. But this wasn't possible in my case. Since I hadn't been in fibrillation before the procedure, it was hard to determine if all the diseased tissue was ablated. Dr. Haïssaguerre said he couldn't verify that he had taken care of all the bad tissue at the right superior pulmonary vein ostium. He also said he had found Atrial Flutter in my right atrium which his colleagues would fix.

Dr. Haïssaguerre went up to see my wife, Patti, to fill her in on what had happened. Meanwhile his colleagues worked on me for another two hours. I felt pain in my right shoulder which they said was normal. They had a lot of problems stopping the flutter in my right atrium in the isthmus between the atrium and the ventricle, possibly because of my two previous ablations. They said they were only able to block the signal in one direction and not the other. They were obviously getting tired. I had been there for over nine hours and was the second person they treated.

Back in my room I was attached to an IV with an anticoagulant, Heparin, dosed out to me automatically to prevent blood clots and stroke. Once I was able, I

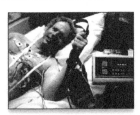

could go to the bathroom and walk around with this IV because it was battery operated when not attached to the wall plug. When this treatment was over, the nurses gave me injections of an anticoagulant in my belly three times a day. I was wiped out and famished at the same time.

I was pretty much out of it Thursday and slept all day. I don't remember much of that day. Friday Dr. Haïssaguerre and Dr. Shah came by to talk to me about what had happened and my prognosis. They

Hooked up in my hospital room in Bordeaux, France

repeated how they weren't sure if they had taken care of all the diseased tissue in the right superior pulmonary vein ostium. They also said they weren't certain they had achieved blockage of my right atrium flutter because of all the previous catheter ablation lines from my first two procedures. They told me they would do a follow-up catheter evaluation of me Wednesday. They suggested that over the weekend, when and if I felt up to it, I should walk up the stairs to see if I could go into A-Fib.

MY A-FIB RETURNS

That weekend I did walk up the stairs and even walked outside in the hospital's park. Sunday, April 26, around 6:15 PM my wife, Patti, and two nurses were in the room with me when I went into A-Fib big time. I felt my heart bounding around, then my pulse speeded up. This was the first time I was ever happy about going into A-Fib. I knew now they could find exactly where the A-Fib was coming from. The nurses got the portable ECG unit and documented my A-Fib. They also had me wear a 12–lead 24–hour battery operated ECG monitor. I didn't come out of the A-Fib attack till around 9:00 PM which was the longest A-Fib attack I had ever had. Monday Dr. Shah said they would do another catheter ablation procedure on me. That night I was going in and out of A-Fib all the time. The nurses felt fortunate to be able to document my attacks, because these ECGs of my A-Fib helped the medical staff pinpoint the source of my A-Fib.

MY SECOND ABLATION

Due to a cancellation, my second catheter ablation procedure was moved up to Tuesday, April 28, at 2:30 PM I went through the same procedure as the week before with different nurses but the same doctors. This time I had no trouble going into A-Fib. Dr. Haïssaguerre later said he just touched the right superior pulmonary vein ostium area and it flew into A-Fib. (After ablation some of the electrical connections may recover, causing the same ablated area to again trigger A-Fib.) Dr. Haïssaguerre said he wound up cauterizing one third of the ostium area. "We try to keep the burns to a minimum," he said. Again he went to see my wife, Patti, to tell her that he felt very good about this procedure, that he thought he had eliminated the focal point A-Fib.

Dr. Shah and a second doctor came in to work on my right atrium to get rid of the atrial flutter. They wound up mapping my whole right atrium. Instead of the normal 20 watts of RF energy, they used 60 watts on me to block the atrial flutter. I didn't even feel it. They said they couldn't use any more RF power without risk of damaging surrounding tissue. Either my isthmus was too thick or the flutter path was too deep to achieve complete blockage. They didn't finish till 8:30 PM.

After they had pulled out the catheters and started to clean me up, I vomited all over the floor. There was blood in the vomit. It looked the color of coffee grounds. The staff thought it might be a sign of ulcers. For some reason this did not bother me at all. I really felt cured of my A-Fib. This vomiting was nothing compared to getting rid of my heart problem.

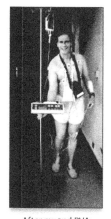

After my 2nd PVA;
Hooked with monitors
and an IV but ambulatory.

The next day, Wednesday, I recovered a lot faster than before. By Thursday I was walking around. Because I had vomited blood, they tested me for ulcers. Again I had to not gag while swallowing a lighted tube that took pictures of my stomach.

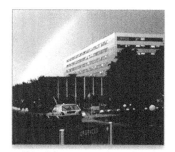

This rainbow appeared over Steve's hospital room the day after his 2nd ablation - we took it as confirmation of his healing; praise God!

They found four little, seemingly new ulcers. Dr. Haïssaguerre and the ulcer doctor thought medication would easily clear these up. These beginning ulcers might have been caused by me not eating since the evening before the procedure, being on anti-coagulants, and/or the strain and length of the operations. As the doctors predicted, once I took the medication, I was cured and haven't felt anything related to ulcers since.

We asked Dr. Haïssaguerre if he could tell from having examined and tested me, what started or caused my A-Fib. He couldn't say for sure. He suggested a viral infection may have started it.

SUCCESS: I'M A-FIB FREE!

I was supposed to stay in the hospital a few more days so that the nurses could give me anti-coagulant shots and monitor the anti-coagulant levels in my blood. But I convinced them I could give myself the anti-coagulant shots in my belly at the right times, and I became an outpatient Friday, May 1, 1998. (Part of my motivation was to save money on hospital costs. I still wound up staying in the hospital 12 days, two more than we had planned.)

MAY 1997: BACK HOME

Once back in the States, I did a follow-up examination with a colleague of Dr. Haïssaguerre's, Dr. Michael Lesh of the University of California at San Francisco Medical Center.

I was A-Fib free! Even though the doctors in France couldn't verify they had fixed the atrial flutter in my right atrium, I didn't have any flutter or fibrillation. I returned to work and felt terrific. The only medication I take is a baby aspirin (81 mg) once a day with breakfast. Annual checkups have revealed no A-Fib symptoms. I resumed my running. I work and train very hard with no apparent side effects.

I feel so fortunate to be free of A-Fib! I thank God for getting me through this and pray I can use the rest of my life to help others with A-Fib.

> ❖ I thank God for getting me through this and pray I can use the rest of my life to help others with A-Fib.

A WEBSITE IS BORN

In 2002, I started a website, *Atrial Fibrillation: Resources for Patients* (*www.A-Fib.com*) written from a patient's point of view, and in plain English, not medicalese. It's my way of passing on to others what I have learned (and will continue to learn) about Atrial Fibrillation. I want to spare others the frustration, depression, and debilitating quality of life the disease caused me.

MINOR A-FIB ATTACK IN 2010

After being free of A-Fib for over twelve years, I had a minor A-Fib attack in September 2010. The symptoms were relatively mild for the most part, but it was noticeable. (I wasn't really surprised and somewhat anticipated it. When I had my ablation back in 1998, they only ablated one of my Pulmonary Veins. Nowadays they routinely ablate all four.)

Because my natural heart rate is so low (48–54 beats/minute from years of running), my doctor was reluctant to put me on meds which might further slow down my heart. We just waited to see if other A-Fib attacks would occur. (I do use the Natural Remedies protocol as a preventive measure as described at A-Fib.com. The only other med I am on is the statin Crestor 10 mg every other day to lower cholesterol.) There was no subsequent episode. Guess it was just a fluke.

2011: THE WEBSITE BIRTHS A BOOK

My website, A-Fib.com started in 2002, has flourished and given birth to a book. I had not expected the need for continued patient education and advocacy. Ten years ago, I had thought that after the FDA approved the Pulmonary Vein Isolation procedure in the U.S. that the need for independent, unbiased patient-focused information would diminish.

Boy! was I wrong.

Just the opposite has happened. Atrial Fibrillation is epidemic among the aging baby-boomer generation. Among the general population, it's predicted to afflict one out of four as they move into their "retirement" years.

Before the widespread use of the web and Internet, there wasn't much information on Atrial Fibrillation available for the layman. And what was found was often out-of-date. Now, we have the opposite situation. Maneuvering the sea of medical information, conflicting opinions, and technical jargon continue to confuse the average A-Fib patient. Who said it? "We are drowning in information and starving for knowledge."[255]

My mission continues—to spare others the frustration, depression, and debilitating quality of life that Atrial Fibrillation caused me.

Steve S. Ryan
Malibu, California, USA

Afterword: It may not be accurate to say that I had three failed ablations before going to Bordeaux, France. It's more precise to say in 1997 I had two catheter ablations of the right atrium, and one aborted attempt of the left atrium. Once in Bordeaux, I had a successful "Focal Point Catheter Ablation" in the left atrium. During my ten-day stay in the hospital, do to recurrence I had a second ablation a week after the first. So does that add up to two failed right atrium ablations and two left-atrium ablations?

Looking back to 1997, I see that the two right atrium ablations were probably a waste of effort for my A-Fib. We know now that A-Fib usually originates in the left atrium. Today, when ablating the left atrium, most EPs will also ablate the right atrium during the same procedure (a two-for-one). This is a precaution against any rogue A-Fib signals originating from the right atrium, as well as to address diagnosed or undiagnosed Atrial Flutter.

Do you have an A-Fib story to share?

Help others by telling your story. We welcome you
to share your own experience with Atrial Fibrillation.
(This includes family members, too.) If you think others
may benefits from reading about your experience with
A-Fib, send us an email to:
DrSteveRyan@BeatYourA-Fib.com, attach your photo
and your story.

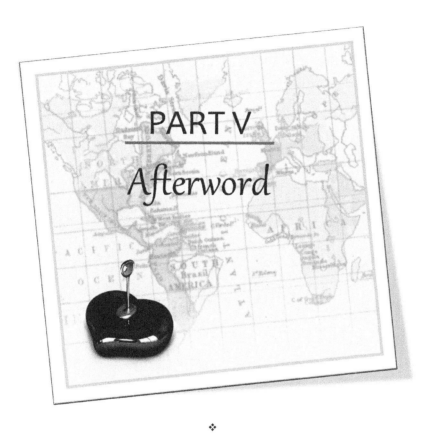

PART V

Afterword

❖

"This story is my testimony... that God is real and he listens to his children's prayers.
I never lost faith in all of this. And I pray that if you are in the shadows of fear,
call on the name of the Lord to give you the light of hope."
Ryan Townsend, Miami, FL
Living with an ICD, but free of A-Fib

❖

Acknowledgements

MY PERSONAL DOCTORS

My special thanks to Drs. Pierre Jaïs and Michel Haïssaguerre of the French Bordeaux group (Hôpital Cardiologique du Haut-Lévêque, France). They changed my life by making me free of A-Fib back in 1998 through a Pulmonary Vein Isolation procedure. Over the years Dr. Jaïs has generously given his time to answer the many questions I have had about A-Fib, and to take care of the many difficult A-Fib cases I have sent him.

In addition to being my personal heart doctors, Dr. Shephal Doshi (St. John's Health Center) and Dr. Walter Kerwin (Cedars-Sinai Medical Center) have also taken the time to answer the many questions I have had about A-Fib. I particularly appreciate Dr. Doshi's effort to make me more safety conscious, leading me to realize that Pulmonary Vein Isolation may not be the best option for everyone. Dr. Kerwin helped me understand the tremendous potential of Cryo and CryoBalloon ablation.

MY RESEARCH AND MEDICAL ADVISORS

I need to thank the many doctors who over the years listened patiently to my many questions and did their best to help me understand basic concepts of A-Fib at the Boston A-Fib Symposium meetings. I especially want to acknowledge Dr. Brian McGovern (Massachusetts General Hospital) who passed away far too soon. I will never forget his warmth and welcoming attitude to a neophyte A-Fib reporter attending his first Boston A-Fib Symposium.

Probably no one else has answered more of my questions than Dr. Jeremy Ruskin (Massachusetts General) who co-organizes the Boston A-Fib Symposiums. The Symposiums have been a tremendous learning experience for me which I've been able to share with other patients. My thanks particularly to Muriel Corcoran (Arrhythmia Education Inc.) who makes sure the Symposiums run smoothly and who has greatly facilitated my efforts.

I'd like to thank the co-directors of the Boston A-Fib Symposiums: Dr. David Keane (St. Vincent's University Hospital, Dublin, Ireland), Dr. Moussa Mansour (Massachusetts General), and Dr. Vivek Reddy (Mount Sinai Medical Center). I'm especially grateful to Dr. Reddy for his many explanations of difficult to understand concepts in A-Fib.

And for their infinite patience in answering my queries, my thanks to: Dr. Hugh Calkins (Johns Hopkins Hospital), Dr. John Camm (St. George's Medical School, London, UK), Dr. Shin-Ann Chen (Veteran's General Hospital, Taiwan), Dr. Ralph Damiano, Jr. (Washington University in St. Louis), Dr. Patrick Ellinor (Mass. General Hospital), Dr. Robert Fishel (Florida Electrophysiology Associates), Dr. Warren Jackman (University of Oklahoma), Dr. Jose Jalife (University of Michigan), Dr. G. Neal Kay (University of Alabama at Birmingham), Dr. Hans Kottkamp (Clinic Hirslanden Heart Center, Switzerland), Dr. David Kress (Midwestern Heart Surgery Institute), Dr. Karl-Heinz Kuck (Asklepios Klinik St Georg, Hamburg, Germany), Dr. Francis Marchlinski (University of Pennsylvania), Dr. Pirooz Mofrad (Washington Heart Rhythm Associates), Dr. Fred Morady (University of Michigan), Dr. Andrea Natale (Texas Cardiac Arrhythmia Inst.), Dr. Stanley Nattel (Montreal Heart

Institute), Dr. Jeffrey E. Olgin (U C San Francisco), Dr. Douglas Packer (Mayo Clinic), Dr. Carlo Pappone (Villa Maria Cecilia Hospital, Italy), Dr. Erik Prystowski (The Care Group), Dr. Dipen Shah (Hopital Cantonal de Geneve, Switzerland), Dr. Wilber Su (Heart Rhythm Specialists of Arizona), Dr. Albert Waldo (University Hospitals of Cleveland), Dr. Marcus Wharton (Medical University of South Carolina), and Dr. David Wilber (Loyola University Medical Center).

Special thanks go to all who read the early drafts of this book and offered suggestions and constructive criticism. I especially want to recognize Karen K. James, Ph.D., for her scholarly review, and for prompting and prodding me when needed, and Dr. Walter Kerwin (Cedars-Sinai Medical Center) for his gracious Foreword, and Dr. Steven C. Hao (California Pacific Medical Center) for his thoughtful Introduction to this book.

MY WEBSITE READERS, VOLUNTEERS, AND CONTRIBUTORS

This book would not be possible without the patients and medical professionals who visit and contribute to my website, *Atrial Fibrillation: Resources for Patients*, better known as *A-Fib.com*. Many offer their ideas, research, and insights to A-Fib.com. In particular, I thank the many people who have contributed their personal experiences in finding their cure. Your stories are probably the most influential and well-read part of A-Fib.com. You give new visitors hope, encouragement, and a sense of what they need to do to deal with their A-Fib.

Thanks to our group of A-Fib support volunteers from the US and around the world who, without being paid, help others get through their A-Fib ordeal. They offer encouragement and caring when needed most. Special thanks goes to Coordinator Nancy Thompson whose enthusiasm and skill keep the program going, and to Joyce Randolph who does such an excellent job organizing meetings and coordinating the local Southern California A-Fib support group. Thanks to Ed Webb for helping get A-Fib.com and our volunteers more involved in social media (Facebook) and who shares his research on A-Fib monitors.

MY FAMILY AND FRIENDS

Thanks to our niece, Julie James, who advised me initially when building the A-Fib.com website in 2002, and who provided invaluable advice on the intricacies of the software; and to Sharion Cox who, in 2010, "freshened up" the look of the website.

I can't thank my wife, Patti, enough for all the effort she has put into this book as editor, and co-writer. She is also the driving force in getting this book done. (She's also the book's graphic designer and publisher; and designed the A-Fib.com logo, too.) She deserves special thanks for always keeping our readers in mind (ordinary folks, not medical personnel), and thereby making the medical information readable, and for not-so-gently steering me away from writing in medical jargon.

❖

About the Authors

Steve Staszak Ryan

Steve had his first A-Fib attack in the January 1997. After much frustration, failed drug therapies, and multiple unsuccessful ablation procedures in the U.S., he educated himself about Atrial Fibrillation through an exhaustive research of medical literature and interviews with medical experts. In April 1998, he was cured in Bordeaux, France, through a then relatively new procedure called Focal Catheter Ablation ("pulmonary Vein Isolation"). He was so grateful for 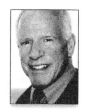 his cure, he pledged to help other A-Fib patients find their cure, too. In 2002, he founded *Atrial Fibrillation: Resources for Patients* (www.A-Fib.com). He continues to research, write, and publish A-Fib.com along with his wife, Patti.

Steve S. Ryan earned a Ph.D. in Educational Communications from the Ohio State University, and for many years taught college level Film (Motion Pictures) Analysis and Television Production. He jumped the fence in 1983, to work in broadcast television at NBC in Burbank, CA. "Retired" in 2001, he devotes most of his time to helping A-Fib patients through A-Fib.com. He's a jogger/sprinter, watches every three and four-star rated movie ever made, and volunteers at church and with the local community emergency response team (CERT).

LinkedIn Profile: Steve S. Ryan, PhD; *Email:* DrSteveRyan@BeatYourA-Fib.com.

Patti James Ryan

When Steve Ryan started planning his website for A-Fib patients, the top priority was presenting timely medical and research information—but in layman's terms, not medicalese. That's where Steve's wife, Patti, enters the picture. With a background in corporate communications, she pledged to fight tooth 'n nail, if needed, to represent the patients' point-of-view and drum out as much medical jargon as possible. And, yes, there were many heated 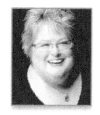 "discussions." Patti also contributes her graphics and photography savvy to A-Fib.com, and BeatYourA–Fib.com.

Patti J. Ryan has a B.F.A. in Fine Art and M.S. in Communications along with university certificates in Business and Corporate Training. Her professional experience includes graphic design, still photography, corporate video production, and business management. In the past few years she has focused on creative project design and writing for the craft and home décor magazine/book publication markets.

LinkedIn profile: Patti J. Ryan; *Email:* PattiJRyan@BeatYourA-Fib.com.

Patti and Steve Ryan have been married for… well, they often relate that they married on the day that Richard Nixon resigned the Presidency of the United States (that's in 1974 for you youngsters). They live in Malibu, California, USA.

❖

Talk with the A-Fib Coach^{SM}

*Steve S. Ryan, PhD
the A-Fib Coach* ^{SM}

Could you use some personal coaching to chart the path to your A-Fib cure? Consider talking one-on-one with Steve S. Ryan, PhD, the A-Fib Coach^{SM}. Steve found his A-Fib cure, and can help you find yours, too.

YOUR SPECIAL DISCOUNT

With the purchase of this book, you're entitled to a discount on your personal one-on-one coaching session. Email us at: A-FibCoach@BeatYourA-Fib.com or visit www.BeatYourA-Fib.com to learn how to apply your book purchase toward your coaching fee.

> *"My consultation with Steve Ryan was extremely helpful. I received excellent advice for my A-Fib condition along with names of reputable doctors to use for my treatment."*
>
> JOE REITMEYER, ELMHURST, IL

ONE-ON-ONE SESSION

Do you need an impartial evaluation of your current A-Fib treatment plan, including medications? Do you want to discuss your needs and treatment options with someone not associated with your medical provider or your health insurance? During your telephone coaching session you can discuss topics such as:

> ➢ The effectiveness (or not) of your current medications
> ➢ Your test results, and which tests you should request
> ➢ Your non-drug treatment options
> ➢ The impact of your other health-related conditions
> ➢ Referrals to electrophysiologists

Your A-Fib Coach^{SM} session is customized to your needs—just send a copy of your personal medical records for Steve to review beforehand. Each session is followed by a personal email from Steve summarizing the key points of your discussion including recommendations and referrals.

For a phone consultation, email Steve Ryan at A-FibCoach@BeatYourA-Fib.com, or visit www.BeatYourA-Fib.com to get more information and rates.

IS YOUR A-FIB MORE COMPLICATED?

Some cases of Atrial Fibrillation are more complicated. Are you facing some difficult choices? Are you dealing with any of the following concerns?

> ➢ Do you have another cardiovascular disease?
> ➢ Do you have a heart valve problem?
> ➢ Have you had heart attacks?
> ➢ Do you have long-standing high blood pressure?

Is your A-Fib concurrent with another health issue?

> ➢ Do you have emphysema?
> ➢ Do you have hyperthyroidism?
> ➢ Do you have diabetes? Or are you significantly overweight?

What A-Fib treatments have you tried?

> Have A-Fib drug therapies been unsuccessful?
> Are you intolerant of the A-Fib medications?
> Have you had one or more ablations that failed?

For a phone consultation, email Steve Ryan at A-FibCoach@BeatYourA-Fib.com, or visit www.BeatYourA-Fib.com to get more information and rates (Discounts are available. No one is turned away for lack of funds.)

> *"Steve has the rare combination of in-depth knowledge and genuine kindness. He has been an invaluable and consistent support to me as I have navigated my way through various treatment options. I can wholeheartedly recommend him as an A-Fib coach; you will be most grateful to have him on your side."*
>
> KATHARINE, VANCOUVER, B.C., CANADA

THE *A-FIB COACH* ^{SM} CAN BE YOUR PATIENT ADVOCATE

You need a well-informed patient advocate who can discuss all your available options, someone who will offer you up-to-date information and unbiased advice.

For over ten years, Dr. Steve Ryan, PhD, has been helping thousands every month through his website, www.A-Fib.com, and through one-on-one counseling directly with A-Fib patients—many who are now free of the burden of Atrial Fibrillation. He found his own cure for A-Fib, and can help you find yours.

For your personal one-on-one coaching session, contact Steve Ryan, the A-Fib Coach[SM]. Email or visit our website, BeatYourA-Fib.com for more information.

YOUR DISCOUNT TOWARD ONE-ON-ONE COACHING

With the purchase of this book, you're entitled to a discount on your personal one-on-one coaching session. Email us at: A-FibCoach@BeatYourA-Fib.com or visit www.BeatYourA-Fib.com to learn how to apply your book purchase toward your coaching fee. (Other discounts are available. No one is turned away for lack of funds.)

❖ 100% Money Back Satisfaction Guarantee ❖

(What have you got to lose, except your A-Fib?)

> *"I have used the A-Fib Coach service on a number of occasions. It is extremely reassuring to have someone who knows the field inside-out take the time to really listen to you and then give helpful advice. It is also reassuring to have this service easily available."*
>
> DAVID HOLZMAN, LEXINGTON MA

Credits: Graphics and Photos

Many generous organizations donated image services, graphics and photos for use in this publication, often from their own patient resources websites. We thank them for contributing to our efforts to educate patients with atrial fibrillation.

Visual 1:   The Cardiac Cycle.
              Figure produced using Servier Medical Art. Used with permission.
Visual 2:   Veins leading to heart.
              Figure produced using Servier Medical Art. Used with permission.
Visual 3:   *Chart:* Percentage of patients with these symptoms (patients could have multiple symptoms).
              © 2011 Patti J. Ryan and A-Fib, Inc.
Visual 4:   ECG strip of heart in normal sinus rhythm.
              © 2011 Patti J. Ryan and A-Fib, Inc.
Visual 5:   ECG strip of a heart in Atrial Fibrillation.
              © 2011 Patti J. Ryan and A-Fib, Inc.
Visual 6:   Heart ventricles and atria.
              © Boston Scientific Corporation. Used with permission.
Visual 7:   ECG strip of Atrial Flutter (with the characteristic saw-tooth pattern).
              © 2011 Patti J. Ryan and A-Fib, Inc.
Visual 8:   How a stroke can occur during Atrial Fibrillation.
              Public domain image. Source: National Institutes of Health.
Visual 9:   (L) The Watchman LAA Closure Device from Atritech.
              © Atritech, Inc. Used with permission.
              (R) Lariat Remote Suture device from SentreHeart.
              © SentreHEART, Inc. Used with permission.
Visual 10:   *Chart:* Prevalence of Atrial Fibrillation in Women and Men by Age Groups.
              © 2011 Patti J. Ryan and A-Fib, Inc.
Visual 11:   Normal 12 lead ECG trace with rhythm strip at the bottom.
              Project IVLine. Used with permission.
Visual 12:   DigiCardioHolter monitor.
              © DigiCardio, Inc. Used with permission.
Visual 13:   Cardionet chestplate Event Monitor: held directly to the chest to make recordings.
              © Cardionet, Inc. Used with permission.
Visual 14:   Medtronic Reveal® DX Implantable monitor.
              © Medtronic, Inc. Used with permission.
Visual 15:   Stress Test System from CardiacScience.
              © CardiacScience. Used with permission.
Visual 16:   Electrophysiology lab.
              © Philips Healthcare. Used with permission.
Visual 17:   Ultrasound equipment.
              © Atlantic Health System. Photographer: Richard Titus. Used with permission.
Visual 18:   Transesophageal Echocardiography.
              © Texas Heart Institute. Used with permission.

Visual 19:   CT Scan procedure rooms.
                © Texas Heart Institute. Used with permission.
Visual 20:   *Table:* Key electrolytes for heart health; Blood serum & intracellular
                electrolyte concentrations for magnesium, calcium and potassium.
Visual 21:   *Table:* Recommended daily minimum or intake for healthy adults;
                Recommended daily supplement dosage of magnesium, calium and
                potassium for A-Fib patients.
Visual 22:   Left Atrial Appendage with catheter placing Watchman device.
                © Atritech.net. Used with permission.
Visual 23:   ECG of A-Fib before and after cardioversion.
                © 2011 Patti J. Ryan and A-Fib, Inc.
Visual 24:   The Pulmonary Circuit. Oxygen-rich blood flows into the heart;
                oxygen-depleted blood flows out.
                Public domain. Source: Wikipedia public domain image.
Visual 25:   (L) Catheter inserted through groin or wrist.
                © University of Ottawa Heart Institute. Used with permission.
                (R) Catheter advanced through septum (wall) into left atrium.
                © BiosenseWebster, Inc. Used with permission.
Visual 26:   The image on the left is taken with X-rays (fluoroscopy). Several
                catheters are seen in the heart. When the CT image is added to the
                frame (shown at the right), the location of the pulmonary veins can
                be clearly identified.
                © Aurora St. Luke's Medical Center/EP Lab. Dr. Jasbir Sra and David
                Krum. Used with permission.
Visual 27:   Catheters create circular ablation lines around each pulmonary vein
                opening.
                © Arquivos Brasileiros de Cardiologia. Used with permission.
Visual 28:   Pulmonary Vein Potentials. (L) Initial electrogram measurements
                show PV potentials (R) Post-therapy all PV potentials eliminated.
                © BiosenseWebster, Inc. Used with permission.
Visual 29:   Arctic Front® Cardiac CryoAblation Catheter by Medtronic (L)
                Closed; (C) Inflate and Position; (R) Occlude and Ablate.
                © Medtronic, Inc. Used with permission.
Visual 30:   (L) Radio Frequency (RF) catheter.
                © BiosenseWebster, Inc. Used with permission.
                (R) Cryo tip removes heat (rather than adding cold).
                © Medtronic, Inc. Used with permission.
Visual 31:   (L) ThermoCool irrigated tip catheter.
                © BiosenseWebster, Inc. Used with permission.
                (C) LASSO 2515 Variable Circular Mapping catheter.
                © BiosenseWebster, Inc. Used with permission.
                (R) CardioFocus balloon catheter steerable sheath.
                © CardioFocus, Inc. Used with permission.
Visual 32:   Sinus Node (SA) and AV Node.
                © Boston Scientific Corporation. Used with permission.
Visual 33:   Surgical Maze pattern of lesions.
                © Nature Publishing Group; Used with permission.

Visual 34:   Maze surgery pattern of RF lesions.
               © Washington University School of Medicine, St. Louis. Used with permission.
Visual 35:   Mini-maze closed chest incisions.
               © 2011 Patti J. Ryan and A-Fib, Inc.
Visual 36:   Internal cardioverter defibrillator (ICD) vs. Pacemaker.
               Public domain image. Source: National Institutes of Health.
Visual 37:   "Finding a Specialist" on the Heart Rhythm Society website.
               © Heart Rhythm Society. Used with permission.

Bibliography

REFERENCES

Abdon, N. J., Zettervall, O., Carlson, J. et al. (1982). Is occult atrial disorder a frequent cause of non-hemorrhagic stroke? Long-term ECG in 86 patients. Stroke, 13 (6), 832-837. Retrieved July 30, 2011, from http://stroke.ahajournals.org/content/13/6/832.abstract

ACC/AHA pocket guideline based on the ACC/AHA/ESC guidelines for the management of patients with atrial fibrillation management of patients with atrial fibrillation. July 2007. Retrieved July 30, 2011 from http://www.af-ablation.org/uploads/Management-of-Patients-with-atrial-fibrillation-pocket.pdf

Adán, V., & Crown, L. A. (2003). Diagnosis and treatment of sick sinus syndrome. American family physician, 67 (8), 1725-1732. Retrieved August 12, 2011, from http://view.ncbi.nlm.nih.gov/pubmed/12725451

Al-Saady, N. M., Obel, O. A., & Camm, A. J. (1999). Left atrial appendage: structure, function, and role in thromboembolism. Heart (British Cardiac Society), 82 (5), 547-554 doi:10.1136/hrt.82.5.547 Retrieved September 12, 2011 from http://heart.bmj.com/content/82/5/547.short

Answering your questions about the electrophysiology study. St. Paul, MN: Boston Scientific, 2008. Cardiac Rhythm Management. C1-196-0808. p 10. Retrieved July 31, 2011, from http://www.bostonscientific.com/lifebeat-online/assets/pdfs/resources/C1-196_0808_EPSPatientBroch.pdf.

Appel, L. J. (chair). (2004). Dietary reference intakes for water, potassium, sodium, chloride, and sulfate. Consensus report. Panel on dietary reference intakes for electrolytes and water. The National Academies Press. Retrieved July 31, 2011, from http://books.nap.edu/openbook.php?record_id=10925

ASA Plavix feasibility study with watchman left atrial appendage closure technology. 2009. ClinicalTrials.gov. Retrieved July 30, 2011, from http://clinicaltrials.gov/ct2/show/NCT00851578

Atrial Fibrillation. InteliHealth: (2008). Medical content reviewed by the faulty of Harvard Medical School. Retrieved July 31, 2011, from http://www.intelihealth.com/IH/ihtIH/WSIHW000/9339/23923.html

AtriCure's AtriClip system receives FDA 510(k) clearance. Press release. June 14, 2010. Retrieved August 16, 2011 from http://www.theheart.org/article/1089215.do

Barclay, L. (2005). Caffeine not associated with increased risk of atrial Fibrillation. Medscape News Today. Retrieved July 31, 2011, from http://www.medscape.com/viewarticle/501279?src=search%29

Bartus, K., Bednarek, J., & Myc, J. et al. (2010). Feasibility of closed-chest ligation of the left atrial appendage in Humans. Heart Rhythm, 8(2), 188-193. URL http://dx.doi.org/10.1016/j.hrthm.2010.10.040

Berkelhammer, C., & Bear, R. A. (1985). A clinical approach to common electrolyte problems: 4. hypomagnesemia. Canadian Medical Association journal, 132 (4), 360-368. Retrieved July 31, 2011 from http://www.ncbi.nlm.nih.gov/pmc/articles/PMC1345822/

Blackshear, J. L., & Odell, J. A. (1985). Appendage obliteration to reduce stroke in cardiac surgical patients with atrial fibrillation. The Annals of thoracic surgery, 61 (2), 755-759. URL http://dx.doi.org/10.1016/0003-4975(95)00887-X

Brown, M. T., & Bussell, J. K. (2011). Medication adherence: WHO cares? Mayo Clinic proceedings. Mayo Clinic , 86 (4), 304-314. URL http://dx.doi.org/10.4065/mcp.2010.0575

Bucerius, J., Gummert, J. F., Borger, M. A., et al. (2003). Stroke after cardiac surgery: a risk factor analysis of 16,184 consecutive adult patients. Ann Thorac Surg, 75 (2), 472-478. Retrieved July 30, 2011, from http://ats.ctsnetjournals.org/cgi/content/abstract/75/2/472

Bunch, T. J., Weiss, J. P., Crandall, B. G., et al. (2010). Atrial fibrillation is independently associated with senile, vascular, and alzheimer's dementia. Heart Rhythm, 7 (4), 433-437. URL http://dx.doi.org/10.1016/j.hrthm.2009.12.004

Burgess, J. (2010). The strategy–what metabolic cardiology means to Afibbers. The AFIB Report, Hans R. Larsen, Editor. Retrieved July 30, 2011, from http://afibbers.org/resources/strategy.pdf

Calkins, H., & Berger, R. (2011) Johns Hopkins special reports: atrial fibrillation: the latest management strategies. ePub.

Calkins, H., Brugada, J., & Packer, D. L. et al. (2007). HRS/EHRA/ECAS expert Consensus Statement on catheter and surgical ablation of atrial fibrillation: recommendations for personnel, policy, procedures and follow-up. A report of the Heart Rhythm Society (HRS) Task Force on catheter and surgical ablation of atrial fibrillation. VII Outcomes and efficacy of catheter ablation of atrial fibrillation. *Europace*, 9, 335-379. URL http://dx.doi.org/10.1093/europace/eun341

Camm, A. J., Kirchhof, P., & Lip, G. Y. et al. (2010). Guidelines for the management of atrial fibrillation: The task force for the management of atrial fibrillation of the european society of cardiology (ESC). European Heart Journal, 31 (19), 2369-2429. URL http://dx.doi.org/10.1093/eurheartj/ehq278

Cannom, D. S. (2000). Atrial fibrillation: nonpharmacologic approaches. American Journal of Cardiology, 85(10), 1, 25-35. Retrieved July 31, 2011 from http://www.ajconline.org/article/S0002-9149(00)00904-8/abstract

Cappato, R., Calkins, H., & Chen, S.-A. (2010). Updated worldwide survey on the methods, efficacy, and safety of catheter ablation for human atrial fibrillation / CLINICAL PERSPECTIVE. Circulation: Arrhythmia and Electrophysiology , 3 (1), 32-38. URL http://dx.doi.org/10.1161/CIRCEP.109.859116

Cardiovascular disease comprehensive 6–other connections: the link between infections and inflammation in heart disease. Life Extension Vitamins. Retrieved July 30, 2011, from http://www.lifeextensionvitamins.com/cadico6otco.html

Cardiovascular disease comprehensive 8 - therapeutic C. Life Extension Vitamins. Retrieved July 30, 2011, from http://www.lifeextensionvitamins.com/cadico8thc.html

Chatterjee, S., Alexander, J. C., Pearson, P. J., & Feldman, T. (2011). Left atrial appendage occlusion: Lessons learned from surgical and transcatheter experiences. *Ann Thorac Surg* , 92 (6), 2283-2292. URL http://dx.doi.org/10.1016/j.athoracsur.2011.08.044

Ciaccio, E. J., Biviano, A. B., Whang, W. et al. (2010). Different characteristics of complex fractionated atrial electrograms in acute paroxysmal versus long-standing persistent atrial fibrillation. Heart rhythm, 7 (9), 1207-1215. URL http://dx.doi.org/10.1016/j.hrthm.2010.06.018

Cohen, Todd J. A patient's guide to heart rhythm problems. Baltimore: Johns Hopkins UP, 2010. 171-72. Print.

Daccarett, M., Badger, T. J., Akoum, N., Burgon, N. S., et al. (2011). Association of left atrial fibrosis detected by Delayed-Enhancement magnetic resonance imaging and the risk of stroke in patients with atrial fibrillation. J Am Coll Cardiol , 57 (7), 831-838. URL http://dx.doi.org/10.1016/j.jacc.2010.09.049

Damiano, R. J. (2008). What is the best way to surgically eliminate the left atrial appendage? Journal of the American College of Cardiology, 52 (11), 930-931. URL http://dx.doi.org/10.1016/j.jacc.2008.06.007

Davis, W. (2007, February). Magnesium Deficiency: Is Your Bottled Water Killing You? Life Extension Magazine. Retrieved September 12, 2011, from http://www.lef.org/magazine/mag2007/feb2007_report_water_01.htm

Dean, Carol. The Magnesium Miracle. 2007. Ballantine Books.

Damiano, R. J., & Bailey, M. (2007). The Cox-Maze IV procedure for lone atrial fibrillation. MMCTS , 2007 (0723), 2758+. URL http://dx.doi.org/10.1510/mmcts.2007.002758

Damiano, R. J., Gaynor, S. L., Bailey, M. et al. (2003). The long-term outcome of patients with coronary disease and atrial fibrillation undergoing the Cox-Maze procedure. The Journal of thoracic and cardiovascular surgery, 126 (6), 2016-2021. URL http://dx.doi.org/10.1016/j.jtcvs.2003.07.006

Damiano, R. J. (2008, February 15). The Cox-Maze IV Procedure: Operative Technique and Results. Slide set. Presented at First Crossing Borders AF Meeting in Netherlands, Maastricht. Retrieved August 22, 2011 from http://www.crossing-borders.info/presentaties/damiano.pdf.

Dell'Orfano, J. T., Luck, J. C., Wolbrette, D. L., Patel, H., & Naccarelli, G. V. (1998). Drugs for conversion of atrial fibrillation. American family physician, 58 (2), 471-480. Retrived Nov. 19, 2011. URL http://view.ncbi.nlm.nih.gov/pubmed/9713400

Dietary Reference Intakes for Calcium and Vitamin D: Report Brief. Revised March 2011, Institute of Medicine of the National Academies. Retrieved August 31, 2011. URL http://www.iom.edu/Reports/2010/Dietary-Reference-Intakes-for-Calcium-and-Vitamin-D.aspx

Dietary Reference Intake (DRI) system. Institute of Medicine (IOM) of the U.S. National Academy of Sciences; Retrieved August 16, 2011 from http://www.cnpp.usda.gov/Publications/DietaryGuidelines/2010/PolicyDoc/Appendices.pdf

Digital Object Identifier System. URL http://www.doi.org/index.html

Drug treatment for atrial fibrillation. 2011. The London Atrial Fibrillation Centre. Retrieved July 31, 2011, from http://www.londonafcentre.co.uk/atrial_fibrillation_treatmentdrugs_for_af

Edgerton, J. R., McClelland, J. H., Duke, D. et al. (2009). Minimally invasive surgical ablation of atrial fibrillation: six-month results. The Journal of thoracic and cardiovascular surgery, 138 (1). URL http://dx.doi.org/10.1016/j.jtcvs.2008.09.080

Electrolyte Imbalance - Normal Adult Values. 2005. Chemo Care. Content provided by Cleveland Clinic Cancer Center. Retrieved August 19, 2011, from http://www.chemocare.com/managing/electrolyte_imbalance.asp

Elias, M. F., Sullivan, L. M., Elias, P. K. et al. (2006). Atrial fibrillation is associated with lower cognitive performance in the framingham offspring men. Journal of stroke and cerebrovascular diseases, 15 (5), 214-222. URL http://dx.doi.org/10.1016/j.jstrokecerebrovasdis.2006.05.009

Evaluation of the Watchman LAA Closure Device in Patients With Atrial Fibrillation Versus Long Term Warfarin Therapy (PREVAIL) 2010. ClinicalTrials.gov. Retrieved July 30, 2011, from http://clinicaltrials.gov/ct2/show/NCT01182441?term=Watchman

EXAtest sample report; Retrieved August 16, 2011 from http://www.exatest.com/PDF%20Files/report1.jpg

Falk, R. H. (2001). Atrial fibrillation. New England Journal of Medicine, 344 (14), 1067-1078. URL http://dx.doi.org/10.1056/NEJM200104053441407

FDA approves first cryoballoon to treat AF. (2010, December 20). Theheart.org by WebMD. Retrieved July 31, 2011, from http://www.bostonscientific.com/lifebeat-online/assets/pdfs/resources/C1-196_0808_EPSPatientBroch.pdf

Feinberg, W. M., Blackshear, J. L., Laupacis, A., et al. (1995). Prevalence, age distribution, and gender of patients with atrial fibrillation. analysis and implications. Archives of internal medicine, 155 (5), 469-473. PubMed PMID: 7864703. Retrieved September 12, 2011 from http://www.ncbi.nlm.nih.gov/pubmed/7864703

Feinberg, W. M., Seeger, J. F., Carmody, R. F., et al. (1990). Epidemiologic features of asymptomatic cerebral infarction in patients with nonvalvular atrial fibrillation. Archives of internal medicine, 150 (11), 2340-2344. Retrieved September 11, 2011 from http://archinte.ama-assn.org/cgi/content/abstract/150/11/2340

Frost, L., & Vestergaard, P. (2005). Caffeine and risk of atrial fibrillation or flutter: the danish diet, cancer, and health study. The American Journal of Clinical Nutrition, 81 (3), 578-582. Retrieved July 30, 2011 from http://www.ajcn.org/content/81/3/578.abstract

Frost, L., Mølgaard, H., Christiansen, E. H. et al. (1992). Atrial fibrillation and flutter after coronary artery bypass surgery: epidemiology, risk factors and preventive trials.

International journal of cardiology, 36 (3), 253-261. Retrieved July 30, 2011 from http://view.ncbi.nlm.nih.gov/pubmed/1358829

Furberg, C. (1994). Prevalence of atrial fibrillation in elderly subjects (the cardiovascular health study). The American Journal of Cardiology, 74 (3), 236-241. URL http://dx.doi.org/10.1016/0002-9149(94)90363-8

Fuster, V., Rydén, L. E., Cannom, D. S. et al. (2006). ACC/AHA/ESC 2006 guidelines for the management of patients with atrial fibrillation—executive summary. Circulation, 114(7), 700–752. URL http://dx.doi.org/10.1161/Circulationaha.106.177031

Ganz, L. I. (2011). Patient information: atrial fibrillation/atrial fibrillation causes. UpToDate Inc. Retrieved July 30, 2011 from http://www.uptodate.com/contents/patient-information-atrial-fibrillation#H

Gillinov, A. M., Blackstone, E. H., & McCarthy, P. M. (2002). Atrial fibrillation: current surgical options and their assessment. Ann Thorac Surg , 74 (6), 2210-2217. Retrieved September 3, 2011 from URL http://ats.ctsnetjournals.org/cgi/content/abstract/74/6/2210

Go, A. S., Hylek, E. M., & Chang, Y. et al. (2001). Prevalence of diagnosed atrial fibrillation in adults: national implications for rhythm management and stroke prevention: the anticoagulation and risk factors in atrial fibrillation (ATRIA) study. Journal of the American Medical Association, 285(18), 2370-2375. URL http://dx.doi.org/10.1001/jama.285.18.2370

Gonzalez, A. (July 07, 2011.). Atrial fibrillation is emerging as the new epidemic. Cardiac Rhythm News. Retrieved August 23, 2011, from http://www.cxvascular.com/crn-latest-news/cardiac-rhythm-news—latest-news/atrial-fibrillation-is-emerging-as-the-new-epidemic

Gupta, D. Atrial fibrillation: which treatment strategy? Ablation or drugs? HeartRhythmSpecialist.co.uk. Retrieved July 31, 2011, from http://www.heartrhythmspecialist.co.uk/Heartrhythmspecialist.co.uk/AF__Ablation_or_drugs.html

Haines, D. E. Atrial fibrillation: new approaches in management, presented by Dr. David Haines. (1999, August 10). [Transcript, Television broadcast]. University of Virginia School of Medicine. Retrieved July 31, 2011 from http://www.A-Fib.com/HainesUnOfVirginiaAtrialFibrillation.htm

Haïssaguerre, M., Hocini, M., & Sanders, P. (2005). Catheter ablation of long-lasting persistent atrial fibrillation: clinical outcome and mechanisms of subsequent arrhythmias. Journal of cardiovascular electrophysiology, 16 (11), 1138-1147. URL http://dx.doi.org/10.1111/j.1540-8167.2005.00308.x

Haïssaguerre, M., Jaïs, P., Shah, D. C. et al. (2000). Electrophysiological end point for catheter ablation of atrial fibrillation initiated from multiple pulmonary venous foci. Circulation, 101 (12), 1409-1417. Retrieved August 01, 2011, from http://view.ncbi.nlm.nih.gov/pubmed/10736285

Haïssaguerre, M., Jaïs, P., Shah, D. C. et al. (1998). Spontaneous initiation of atrial fibrillation by ectopic beats originating in the pulmonary veins. The New England journal of medicine, 339 (10), 659-666. URL http://dx.doi.org/10.1056/NEJM199809033391003

Han, F. T., Kasirajan, V., Kowalski, M., et al. (2009). Results of a minimally invasive surgical pulmonary vein isolation and ganglionic plexi ablation for atrial fibrillation: single-center experience with 12-month follow-up. Circulation. Arrhythmia and electrophysiology, 2 (4), 370-377. URL http://dx.doi.org/10.1161/CIRCEP.109.854828

Health information privacy. United States Department of Health and Human Services. Retrieved August 01, 2011, from http://www.hhs.gov/ocr/privacy/

HeartScape: The chambers of the heart. 2005. SkillStat Learning. Retrieved July 30, 2011, from http://www.skillstat.com/heartscape/chambers.htm

Heeringa, J., Kors, J. A., & Hofman, A. (2008). Cigarette smoking and risk of atrial fibrillation: the Rotterdam study. American heart journal , 156 (6), 1163-1169. URL http://dx.doi.org/10.1016/j.ahj.2008.08.003

Hondo, T., Okamoto, M., Yamane, T., et al. (1995). The role of the left atrial appendage. a volume loading study in open-chest dogs. Japanese heart journal, 36 (2), 225-234. Retrieved July 31, 2011 from http://view.ncbi.nlm.nih.gov/pubmed/7596042

Hughes, S. (2010, June 18). AtriClip for left atrial appendage occlusion approved in US. Theheart.org. Retrieved August 15, 2011, from http://www.theheart.org/article/1089215.do

Jais, P. Improved A-Fib Procedure. Summary of peer presentation. North American Society of Pacing and Electrophysiology Convention (NASPE), San Diego, CA May, 2002, San Diego. Retrieved July 31, 2011 from http://www.A-Fib.com/HeartRhythmSociety2002.htm

Jaïs, P., Weerasooriya, R., Shah, D. C. et al. (2002). Ablation therapy for atrial fibrillation (AF): past, present and future. Cardiovascular Research, 54 (2), 337-346. URL http://dx.doi.org/10.1016/S0008-6363(02)00263-8

Kääb, S. (2010, February). When the heart gets out of step: Newly identified gene may open route to innovative treatments for atrial fibrillation. LMU Munich. Retrieved August 27, 2011, from http://www.en.uni-muenchen.de/news/newsarchiv/2010/2010-kaab.html

Karjalainen, J., Kujala, U. M., & Kaprio, J. et al. (1998). Lone atrial fibrillation in vigorously exercising middle aged men: case-control study. BMJ (Clinical research ed.), 316 (7147), 1784-1785. Retrieved August 01, 2011, from http://www.ncbi.nlm.nih.gov/pmc/articles/PMC28577/

Katan, M. B., & Schouten, E. (2005). Caffeine and arrhythmia. The American Journal of Clinical Nutrition, 81 (3), 539-540. Retrieved July 30, 2011 from http://www.ajcn.org/content/81/3/539.abstract

Katkhouda, N., Mason, R. J., Towfigh, S., et al. (2005). Laparoscopic versus open appendectomy: a prospective randomized double-blind study. Annals of surgery, 242 (3). Retrieved Nov 30, 2011. URL http://www.ncbi.nlm.nih.gov/pmc/articles/PMC1357752/

Kim, M. H., Johnston, S. S., Chu, B.-C., Dalal, M. R., & Schulman, K. L. (2011). Estimation of total incremental health care costs in patients with atrial fibrillation in the united states. Circulation: Cardiovascular Quality and Outcomes . URL http://dx.doi.org/10.1161/CIRCOUTCOMES.110.958165

King, D. E., Mainous, A. G., Geesey, M. E., et al. (2005). Dietary magnesium and c-reactive protein levels. Journal of the American College of Nutrition, 24 (3), 166-171. URL http://www.jacn.org/cgi/content/abstract/24/3/166

Kiser, A. C., & Mounsey, P. (2009). Convergent Procedure A Total Solution: The atrial fibrillation (AF) population is growing. UNC Cardiac Surgery and Electrophysiology Services. Retrieved July 29, 2011, from http://www.uncheartandvascular.org/index.php?d=7&p=106

Knox, K. (2008). An atrial fibrillation cause that you haven't been told.... Easy Immune System Health. Retrieved July 31, 2011, from http://www.easy-immune-health.com/atrial-fibrillation-cause.html

Kodama, S., Saito, K., & Tanaka, S. et al. (2011). Alcohol consumption and risk of atrial fibrillation: A Meta-Analysis. J Am Coll Cardiol , 57 (4), 427-436. Retrieved Nov. 19, 2011. URL http://dx.doi.org/10.1016/j.jacc.2010.08.641

Kron, J., Kasirajan, V., Wood, M. A., et al. (2010). Management of recurrent atrial arrhythmias after minimally invasive surgical pulmonary vein isolation and ganglionic plexi ablation for atrial fibrillation. Heart rhythm, 7 (4), 445-451. URL http://dx.doi.org/10.1016/j.hrthm.2009.12.008

Kuck, K. H. Five-year follow-up of catheter ablation for PAF. Summary of peer presentation. Boston Atrial Fibrillation Symposium, Boston, MA. January, 14, 2011. Retrieved July 31, 2011 from http://www.A-Fib.com/BostonA-FibSymposium2011.htm

Kühne, M., Schaer, B., Ammann, P., et al. (2010). Cryoballoon ablation for pulmonary vein isolation in patients with paroxysmal atrial fibrillation. Swiss Med Wkly. 2010 Apr 17;140 (15-16), 214-221. Abstract. PubMed PMID:20407957

Kunz, J. S., Hemann, B., Edwin Atwood, J., et al. (2010). Is there a link between gastroesophageal reflux disease and atrial fibrillation? Clin Cardiol, 32 (10), 584-587. URL http://dx.doi.org/10.1002/clc.20660

Lall, S. C., Melby, S. J., Voeller, R. K. et al. (2007). The effect of ablation technology on surgical outcomes after the Cox-Maze procedure: A propensity analysis. J Thorac Cardiovasc Surg, 133 (2), 389-396. URL http://dx.doi.org/10.1016/j.jtcvs.2006.10.009

Lane, D. A., Langman, C. M., Lip, G. Y., & Nouwen, A. (2009). Illness perceptions, affective response, and health-related quality of life in patients with atrial fibrillation. Journal of psychosomatic research , 66 (3), 203-210. URL http://dx.doi.org/10.1016/j.jpsychores.2008.10.007

Larsen, H. R. Flutter ablation may unmask AF. The AFIB Report, 2010. 103, 6-7. Retrieved July 31, 2011, from http://www.afibbers.org/afib103jh.pdf

Lazarides, L. Laboratory Tests for Nutritional Deficiencies. Health-Diets.Net: Nutrition Information and Resources from Linda Lazarides. Adapted from the Nutritional Health Bible by Linda Lazarides, 1998. Retrieved August 21, 2011, from http://www.health-diets.net/healthsearch/nutritionaldeftests.htm

Lin, W.-S. S., Tai, C.-T. T., & Hsieh, M.-H. H. et al. (2003). Catheter ablation of paroxysmal atrial fibrillation initiated by non-pulmonary vein ectopy. Circulation , 107 (25), 3176-3183. URL http://dx.doi.org/10.1161/01.CIR.0000074206.52056.2D

Lloyd-Jones, D. M. (2004). Beyond the numbers: epidemiology and treatment of atrial fibrillation. Medscape Education. Retrieved July 30, 2011, from http://www.medscape.org/viewarticle/494006_2

Loftus, B. D. (2002). Atrial fibrillation and stroke. Bellaire Neurology. Retrieved July 29, 2011, from http://www.loftusmd.com/Articles/stroke/atrialfibrillation.html

Longoria, J. (2010, July 22). Methods of treating a cardiac arrhythmia by thoracoscopic production of a Cox-Maze III lesion set. Patent application. *PatentDocs*. Retrieved Aug. 5, 2011 from http://www.faqs.org/patents/app/20100185186

Longoria, J. and Wolff, L. Totally thoracoscopic epicardial RF ablation for atrial fibrillation using Atricure minimally invasive products. [Transcript, Television broadcast]. (2007, July 24). Sacramento, CA: ORLive.com. Retrieved August 5, 2011, from http://www.or-live.com/transcripts/2007/atr_1822_610.pdf

Lubitz, S. A., Yin, X., Fontes, J. D. et al. (2010). Association between familial atrial fibrillation and risk of new-onset atrial fibrillation. JAMA. 304 (20), 2263-2269. URL http://dx.doi.org/10.1001/jama.2010.1690

Ludwig-Maximilians-Universität München. (2010).When the heart gets out of step: Newly identified gene may open route to innovative treatments for atrial fibrillation Press release. Retrieved July 30, 2011 from http://www.eurekalert.org/pub_releases/2010-02/lm-wth021910.php

Maisel, W. H., Rawn, J. D., & Stevenson, W. G. (2001). Atrial fibrillation after cardiac surgery. Annals of internal medicine, 135 (12), 1061-1073. URL http://view.ncbi.nlm.nih.gov/pubmed/11747385

Marchlinski, F. Pulmonary Vein Isolation Alone for Long Standing Persistent A-Fib. Summary of peer presentation. Boston Atrial Fibrillation Symposium, Boston, MA. January, 14, 2011. Retrieved July 31, 2011 from http://www.A-Fib.com/BostonA-FibSymposium2011.htm

Marijon, E., Albenque, J.-P. P., & Boveda, S. (2009). Feasibility and safety of same-day home discharge after radiofrequency catheter ablation. The American journal of cardiology , 104 (2), 254-258. URL http://dx.doi.org/10.1016/j.amjcard.2009.03.024

Maugh, II, T. H. (2010, November 16). New drugs may replace problematic blood thinner. Los Angeles Times, p.A12.

McCabe, P. J. (2010). Psychological distress in patients diagnosed with atrial fibrillation: the state of the science. The Journal of cardiovascular nursing, 25 (1), 40-51. URL http://dx.doi.org/10.1097/JCN.0b013e3181b7be36

McCarthy, J. T., & Kumar, R. Divalent Cation Metabolism: Magnesium, Chapter 4: *Disorders of Water, Electrolytes, and Acid-Base*, Vol. 1. R. W. Schrier (Ed.), 2000. The Atlas of Diseases of the Kidney series). Online chapter retrieved August 20, 2011 at http://www.cybernephrology.ualberta.ca/cn/Schrier/Volume1/chap4/ADK1_4_1-3.PDF

Medifocus guidebook on: atrial fibrillation: a comprehensive guide to symptoms, treatment, research, and support. Medifocus.com, Inc. July 2010. Vol. #CR004. 40. Print.

Metin, G., Yildiz, M., & Bayraktar, B. et al. (2010). Assessment of the P wave dispersion and duration in elite women basketball players. Indian Pacing Electrophysiol J. Retrieved August 01, 2011, from http://www.ncbi.nlm.nih.gov/pmc/articles/PMC2803602/

Minimally-invasive radiofrequency ablation for atrial fibrillation. Johns Hopkins Medicine. Retrieved August 01, 2011, from http://www.hopkinsmedicine.org/heart_vascular_institute/conditions_treatments/treatments/minimally_invasive_radiofrequency_ablation.html

Miyasaka, Y., Barnes, M. E., Gersh, B. J. et al. (2006). Secular Trends in Incidence of Atrial Fibrillation in Olmsted County, Minnesota, 1980 to 2000, and Implications on the Projections for Future Prevalence. Circulation, 114(2) (Epub Jul. 3), 119-125. URL http://dx.doi.org/10.1161/circulationaha.105.595140

Mont, L., Elosua, R., & Brugada, J. (2009). Endurance sport practice as a risk factor for atrial fibrillation and atrial flutter. Europace, 11 (1), 11-17. URL http://dx.doi.org/10.1093/europace/eun289

Mueller, D. K. (2009, June 4). Mediastinitis: Overview/Background. Medscape Reference. Retrieved September 17, 2011, from http://emedicine.medscape.com/article/425308-overview

Nainggolan, L. (2008). Cryoablation: Safer than RF but slightly lower success rate? Theheart.org by WebMD. Retrieved August 1, 2011, from http://www.theheart.org/article/877315.do Natale, A., & Jalife, J. Atrial fibrillation from bench to bedside. Totowa, NJ: Humana Press. 2008. 103-104. Print.

Narumiya, T. et al. "Relationship between left atrial appendage function and left atrial thrombus in patients with nonvalvular chronic atrial fibrillation and atrial flutter." Circ. J 2003 Jan;67(1):68-72. URL http://www.ncbi.nlm.nih.gov/pubmed/12520155

Navarrete, A., Conte, F., Moran, M., Ali, I., & Milikan, N. (2011). Ablation of atrial fibrillation at the time of cavotricuspid isthmus ablation in patients with atrial flutter without documented atrial fibrillation derives a better Long-Term benefit. Journal of Cardiovascular Electrophysiology, 22 (1), 34-38. URL http://dx.doi.org/10.1111/j.1540-8167.2010.01845.x

Open Heart Surgery Complications. (2006, November 1). EMedTV. Retrieved September 17, 2011, from http://heart-disease.emedtv.com/open-heart-surgery/open-heart-surgery-complications-p2.html

O'Riordan, M. (2011, January 5). Sobering long-term outcomes following ablation of atrial fibrillation. Theheart.org. Retrieved August 01, 2011, from http://www.theheart.org/article/1168671.do

O'Riordan, M. (2009). RECORD AF: Better success with rhythm control, but no difference in outcomes. Theheart.org. Retrieved August 01, 2011, from http://www.theheart.org/article/1023939.do

Ouyang, F., Tilz, R., & Chun, J. (2010). Long-Term results of catheter ablation in paroxysmal atrial fibrillation: Lessons from a 5-Year Follow-Up. Circulation, 122 (23), 2368-2377. URL http://dx.doi.org/10.1161/Circulationaha.110.946806

Peykar, S., & Estrada, J. C. (2010). Atrial fibrillation. Cardiac Arrhythmia Institute. Retrieved July 30, 2011, from http://www.caifl.com/atrial-fibrillation.html

Potassium online textbook. University of Tennessee Health Science Center, Division of Nephrology. Retrieved August 20, 2011 from http://www.uthsc.edu/nephrology/documents/potassium-textbook.pdf

Potassium Supplements, Vitamins & Health Supplements Guide. (2005). Retrieved August 20, 2011, from http://www.vitamins-supplements.org/dietary-minerals/potassium.php

Pradaxa. Boehringer Ingelheim Pharmaceuticals Inc. (2010). Full Prescribing Information, Clinical Trials Experience, Gastrointestinal Adverse Reactions. Retrieved July 31, 2011, from http://dailymed.nlm.nih.gov/dailymed/lookup.cfm?setid=ba74e3cd-b06f-4145-b284-5fd6b84ff3c9

Professional answers to your atrial fibrillation questions: what are the risks of AF ablation? Atrial Fibrillation Institute/St. Vincent's HealthCare. Retrieved August 01, 2011, from http://www.afibjax.com/faq.php

Prystowsky, E. N., Benson, D. W., & Fuster, V. et al. (2000). Management of patients with atrial fibrillation: A statement for healthcare professionals from the subcommittee on electrocardiography and electrophysiology, American Heart Association. Circulation, 93 (6), 1262-1277. Retrieved August 9, 2011, from http://circ.ahajournals.org/content/93/6/1262.abstract

Radiofrequency catheter ablation is considered safe. (2010). AFIB Alliance: Atrial Fibrillation Resource. Retrieved August 01, 2011, from http://www.atrialfibrillation.com/medical-prof/therapy-outcome/safety

Reynolds, M., Lavelle, T., & Essebag, V. et al. (2006). Influence of age, sex, and atrial fibrillation recurrence on quality of life outcomes in a population of patients with new-onset atrial fibrillation: The Fibrillation Registry Assessing Costs, Therapies, Adverse events and Lifestyle (FRACTAL) study. American Heart Journal, 152(6), 1097-1103. URL http://dx.doi.org/10.1016/j.ahj.2006.08.011

Romano, M. A., Bach, D. S., & Pagani, F. D. (2004). Atrial reduction plasty Cox-Maze procedure: extended indications for atrial fibrillation surgery. The Annals of thoracic surgery, 77 (4). URL http://dx.doi.org/10.1016/j.athoracsur.2003.06.022

Rutherford David Rogers. American librarian: The New York Public Library (1954-1957); Library of Congress (1957-1964), Stanford University (1964-1969) and Yale University (1969-1985).

Savelieva, I., & Camm, A. J. (2000). Clinical relevance of silent atrial fibrillation: prevalence, prognosis, quality of life, and management. Journal of interventional cardiac, 4 (2), 369-382. Retrieved July 31, 2011 from http://view.ncbi.nlm.nih.gov/pubmed/10936003

Savelieva I, Camm J. Update on atrial fibrillation: part II. Clin Cardiol. 2008 Mar;31(3):102-8. Review. PubMed PMID: 18383050. URL Retrieved Nov 17, 2011. http://www.ncbi.nlm.nih.gov/pubmed?term=PMID%3A%2018383050

Sawhney, N., Anousheh, R., Chen, W.-C. C. et al. (2009). Five-year outcomes after segmental pulmonary vein isolation for paroxysmal atrial fibrillation. The American journal of cardiology, 104 (3), 366-372. URL http://dx.doi.org/10.1016/j.amjcard.2009.03.044

Schaff, H. V., Dearani, J. A., Daly, R. C., et al. (2000). Cox-Maze procedure for atrial fibrillation: Mayo clinic experience. Seminars in thoracic and cardiovascular surgery, 12 (1), 30-37. Retrieved September 14, 2011, from http://view.ncbi.nlm.nih.gov/pubmed/10746920

Scheinman, M. M., & Morady, F. (2001). Nonpharmacological approaches to atrial fibrillation. Circulation, 103 (16), 2120-2125. Retrieved July 31, 2011 from http://circ.ahajournals.org/content/103/16/2120.abstract.

Schoonderwoerd, B. A., Smit, M. D., Pen, L. et al. (2008). New risk factors for atrial fibrillation: causes of 'not-so-lone atrial fibrillation'. Europace, 10 (6), 668-673. URL http://dx.doi.org/10.1093/europace/eun124

Schuchert, A., Behrens, G., & Meinertz, T. (1999). Impact of long-term ECG recording on the detection of paroxysmal atrial fibrillation in patients after an acute ischemic stroke. PACE, 22 (7), 1082-1084. Retrieved July 30, 2011, from http://view.ncbi.nlm.nih.gov/pubmed/10456638

Seelig, M.S., and Rosanoff, A. The Magnesium Factor, 2003. Avery Trade.

Sharma, K. (2011). Calcium to magnesium ratio. Enerex Botanicals Ltd. Retrieved July 31, 2011 from http://www.enerex.ca/en/articles/calcium-to-magnesium-ratio

Siddoway, L. A. (2003). Amiodarone: guidelines for use and monitoring. American family physician, 68 (11), 2189-2196. Retrieved Nov. 19, 2011. URL http://view.ncbi.nlm.nih.gov/pubmed/14677664

Silver, B. B. (2004). Development of cellular magnesium nano-analysis in treatment of clinical magnesium deficiency. Journal of the American College of Nutrition, 23 (6), 732S-737S. Retrieved July 30, 2011, from http://www.jacn.org/content/23/6/732S.abstract

Sinatra, S. T. (2011). Understanding arrhythmias/causes of arrhythmia/electrolyte imbalances. Heart MD Institute. Retrieved August 1, 2011, from http://www.heartmdinstitute.com/health-concerns/cardiovascular-system/heart-health/atrial-fibrillation-other-arrhythmias

Sleep apnea and sleep. National Sleep Foundation. Retrieved July 30, 2011, from http://www.sleepfoundation.org/article/sleep-topics/sleep-apnea-and-sleep

Stengler, M. (2011) Bottom Line Natural Healing. Vol.7, No.9, September 2011.

Stroke Signs and Symptoms. (2011, August 17). UCSF Medical Center. Retrieved September 03, 2011, from http://www.ucsfhealth.org/conditions/stroke/signs_and_symptoms.html

Understanding Arrhythmias: When the Beat Just Isn't Going on As Usual. Dr. Stephen Sinatra's Heart MD Institute,, P.A. Retrieved August 18, 2011 from http://www.heartmdinstitute.com/health-concerns/cardiovascular-system/heart-health/atrial-fibrillation-other-arrhythmias

Van Wagoner, D. R. (2003). Atrial fibrillation and potassium. Common questions and answers/resources for patients/Cleveland Clinic. Retrieved July 31, 2011 from http://my.clevelandclinic.org/heart/askdoctor/afib_potassium.aspx

Van Wagoner, D.R. (2005). Atrial selective strategies for treating atrial fibrillation. Drug Discovery Today: Therapeutic Strategies, 2(3): 291-295, 2005. Print. Abstract retrieved August 24, 2011 from http://pubget.com/paper/pgtmp_fe0042614504d62a4caa12c2a8d96415

Veinot, J. P., Harrity, P. J., Gentile, F. et al. (1997). Anatomy of the normal left atrial appendage: A quantitative study of Age-Related changes in 500 autopsy hearts: Implications for echocardiographic examination. Circulation, 96 (9), 3112-3115. Retrieved September 11, 2011 from http://circ.ahajournals.org/content/96/9/3112.full

Villareal, R. P., Hariharan, R., Liu, B. C., et al. (2004). Postoperative atrial fibrillation and mortality after coronary artery bypass surgery. Journal of the American College of Cardiology , 43 (5), 742-748. URL http://dx.doi.org/10.1016/j.jacc.2003.11.023

Wanahita, N., Messerli, F. H., Bangalore, S. et al. (2008). Atrial fibrillation and obesity-results of a meta-analysis. American heart journal, 155 (2), 310-315. URL http://dx.doi.org/10.1016/j.ahj.2007.10.004

Wells, P. (2008). Wolff-Parkinson-white syndrome/prognosis of WPW. HeartTracings.com. Retrieved August 03, 2011, from http://www.heartracing.com/physicians/wolff-parkinson-white.syndrome.asp

Who is at risk for atrial fibrillation? U.S. Department of Health & Human Services/National Institutes of Health. Retrieved August 1, 2011, from http://www.nhlbi.nih.gov/health/dci/Diseases/af/af_risk.html

Wilber, D. (2011). Very late recurrence after catheter ablation of AF: Incidence and implications. Summary of peer presentation. Boston Atrial Fibrillation Symposium, Boston, MA. January, 14, 2011. Retrieved July 31, 2011 from http://www.A-Fib.com/BostonA-FibSymposium2011.htm

Wolf, P. A., Abbott, R. D., & Kannel, W. B. (1987). Atrial fibrillation: a major contributor to stroke in the elderly. The framingham study. Archives of internal medicine, 147 (9), 1561-1564. Retrieved July 30, 2011 from URL http://view.ncbi.nlm.nih.gov/pubmed/3632164

Wolf, R. K., Schneeberger, E. W., Osterday, R., Miller, D. et al. (2005). Video-assisted bilateral pulmonary vein isolation and left atrial appendage exclusion for atrial fibrillation. The Journal of thoracic and cardiovascular surgery, 130 (3), 797-802. URL http://dx.doi.org/10.1016/j.jtcvs.2005.03.041

Wolf, R. The wolf mini-maze surgery. The Wolf Mini-Maze website. Retrieved July 30, 2011, from http://www.wolfminimaze.com/index3.html

Women & Atrial Fibrillation. Center for Atrial Fibrillation, Northwestern Memorial Hospital. Retrieved July 31, 2011, from http://www.nmh.org/nm/women-and-atrial-fibrillation

Woodard, MD, O. (2009, April 20). Magnesium: Do You Have Enough? Great Health in Tough Times. Retrieved August 21, 2011, from http://otiswoodardmd.typepad.com/my_weblog/2009/04/magnesium-do-you-have-enough.html

Wyndham, C. R. (2000). Atrial fibrillation: the most common arrhythmia. Texas Heart Institute journal /Texas Heart Institute of St. Luke's Episcopal Hospital, Texas Children's Hospital,

27 (3), 257-267. Retrieved August 9, 2011, from
    http://www.ncbi.nlm.nih.gov/pmc/articles/PMC101077/
Wyse, D. G. (1997). Atrial fibrillation: the clinically relevant trials and results. Annual Scientific
    Session of the American College of Cardiology, Anaheim, California. (1997, March).
    Retrieved July 31, 2011, from http://www.pslgroup.com/dg/25f9a.htm
Yamada, T., Murakami, Y., Okada, T. et al. (2008). Electroanatomic mapping in the catheter
    ablation of premature atrial contractions with a non-pulmonary vein origin. Europace, 10
    (11), 1320-1324. URL http://dx.doi.org/10.1093/europace/eun238
Young, T., Palta, M., & Dempsey, J. (1993). The occurrence of sleep-disordered breathing
    among middle-aged adults. New England Journal of Medicine, 1993;328(17):1230-1235.
    Retrieved July 30, 2011
    http://www.nejm.org/doi/full/10.1056/NEJM199304293281704#t=abstract

ONLINE RESOURCES

ABMS Certification Matters: https://www.certificationmatters.org/is-your-doctor-board-
    certified/search-now.aspx
AFAnswers: http://www.afanswers.com/
A-Fibcures–Non-Pharmaceutical Cures for A-Fib: http://health.groups.yahoo.com/group/A-
    Fibcures/
AFIBsupport: http://www.afibbers.org/bulletin.htm
AF-Ideas.com: http://www.af-ideas.com/
Arrhythmia Alliance (UK): http://www.arrhythmiaalliance.org.uk/
Atrial Fibrillation Association–US: http://www.atrialfibrillation-us.org/
Atrial Fibrillation Patients Who Do Not Respond to Antiarrhythmic Drugs Should Be Treated
    With Catheter Ablation:
    http://www.insidermedicine.com/archives/INSIDERMEDICINE_VIDEO_Atrial_Fibrillation
    _Patients_Who_Do_Not_Respond_to_Antiarrhythmic_Drugs_Should_Be_Treated_Wit
    h_Catheter_Ablation_4047.aspx
Atrial Fibrillation: http://www.youtube.com/watch?v=vGojnxVQ7bM
Atrial Fibrillation: The Latest Management Strategies, Calkins and Berger
    http://www.medifocus.com/2009/landing.php?gid=CR004&a=a&assoc=linkshare
Atrial Fibrillation–Resources for Patients: http://www.a-fib.com/DoctorsFacilities.htm
CenterWatch: http://centerwatch.com/
Choosing a Non-Drug Treatment for Atrial Fibrillation: http://www.af-
    ideas.com/Choosing%20treatment%20for%20atrial%20fibrillation.htm
Cleveland Clinic Center for Atrial Fibrillation:
    http://my.clevelandclinic.org/heart/atrial_fibrillation/afib.aspx
ClinicalTrials.gov: http://clinicaltrials.gov/
CryoAblation Balloon Catheter: http://www.cryocath.de/en/4.products/af.presentation.asp
DoYourProxy.org: http://www.doyourproxy.org/webtool.php
Google Alerts: http://www.google.com/alerts?hl=en
Google Scholar: http://scholar.google.com/schhp?hl=en&tab=ws
HealthGrades: http://www.healthgrades.com/
Heart Care Centers of Illinois: http://www.heartcc.com/AFib.htm
Heart Rhythm Society:
    http://www.hrsonline.org/PatientInfo/HeartRhythmDisorders/AFib/index.cfm
How the Healthy Heart Works:
    http://www.youtube.com/watch?v=i9ILX2a1dS8&feature=related
HRS Finding a Doctor: http://www.hrsonline.org/PatientInfo/specialist_locator.cfm
Listen to a Heart: Sound of the heart in A-Fib: http://filer.case.edu/~dck3/heart/sounds/af.wav;
    Normal Heart Beat: http://youtu.be/NeMJXMSkA7g.
London Atrial Fibrillation Centre: http://www.londonafcentre.co.uk/
Lone Atrial Fibrillation Bulletin Board: http://www.afibbers.org/bulletin.htm
Medical Alert I.D. Wallet Card: http://www.medids.com/free-id.php

MediFocus Guidebook on Atrial Fibrillation, Kindle Edition.
　　http://www.medifocus.com/2009/landing.php?gid=CR004&a=a&assoc=linkshare
MedlinePlus/Arrhythmia: http://www.nlm.nih.gov/medlineplus/arrhythmia.html
Medscape Today: http://www.medscape.com/resource/atrialfibrillation
MyConsult Online Medical Second Opinion: http://eclevelandclinic.org/myconsult
Overview of Atrial Fibrillation:
　　http://streamed.wired.md/display2.pl?doc_user=3623&submit_type=play&enter_type=
　　web&resize=615x700&Procedure=V1072&streamtype=fhi&suppressButtons=yes
PubMed/Medline.gov: http://www.ncbi.nlm.nih.gov/pubmed/
Pulmonary vein Isolation Procedure: http://arrhythmia.ucla.edu/body.cfm?id=39
The American Heart Association:
　　http://www.heart.org/HEARTORG/Conditions/Arrhythmia/Arrhythmia_UCM_002013_Su
　　bHomePage.jsp
The Heart Forum: http://www.medhelp.org/forums/Cardio/WWWboard.html
The Stepwise Approach to Interpreting an ECG:
　　http://www.insidermedicine.com/archives/In_the_Clinic_-
　　_Dr_Chris_Simpson_MD_on_the_Stepwise_Approach_to_Interpreting_an_ECG_1800.a
　　spx
UpToDate: http://patients.uptodate.com/topic.asp?file=hrt_dis/4882
Vitals.com: http://www.vitals.com/
Your Rights To Your Medical Records Under HIPAA: http://www.hhs.gov/ocr/privacy/

❖

Note: online destinations and content change without warning. Websites and web
addresses are current as of our publication date.

❖

Endnotes

An extensive list of medical journal articles, research studies, scholarly presentations and other references were used in the writing of this book (and the website www. A-Fib.com). Each footnote reference is included below.

Consult your local public library or university medical school library for help to locate these materials. Many of these documents can be accessed online. We've included websites, hyperlinks, and a Digital Object Identifier (DOI)[256] address when possible.

[1] Kääb, S. (2010, February). When the heart gets out of step: Newly identified gene may open route to innovative treatments for atrial fibrillation. LMU Munich. Retrieved August 27, 2011, from http://www.en.uni-muenchen.de/news/newsarchiv/2010/2010-kaab.html

[2] Kim, M. H., Johnston, S. S., Chu, B.-C., Dalal, M. R., & Schulman, K. L. (2011). Estimation of total incremental health care costs in patients with atrial fibrillation in the United States. Circulation: Cardiovascular Quality and Outcomes . URL http://dx.doi.org/10.1161/CIRCOUTCOMES.110.958165

[3] Miyasaka, Y., Barnes, M. E., Gersh, B. J. et al. (2006). Secular Trends in Incidence of Atrial Fibrillation in Olmsted County, Minnesota, 1980 to 2000, and Implications on the Projections for Future Prevalence. Circulation, 114(2) (Epub Jul. 3), 119-125. URL http://dx.doi.org/10.1161/circulationaha.105.595140

[4] Kiser, A. C., & Mounsey, P. (2009). Convergent Procedure A Total Solution: The atrial fibrillation (AF) population is growing. UNC Cardiac Surgery and Electrophysiology Services. Retrieved July 29, 2011, from http://www.uncheartandvascular.org/index.php?d=7&p=106

[5] Reynolds, M., Lavelle, T., & Essebag, V. et al. (2006). Influence of age, sex, and atrial fibrillation recurrence on quality of life outcomes in a population of patients with new-onset atrial fibrillation: The Fibrillation Registry Assessing Costs, Therapies, Adverse events and Lifestyle (FRACTAL) study. American Heart Journal, 152(6), 1097-1103. URL http://dx.doi.org/10.1016/j.ahj.2006.08.011

[6] Fuster, V., Rydén, L. E., Cannom, D. S. et al. (2006). ACC/AHA/ESC 2006 guidelines for the management of patients with atrial fibrillation—executive summary. Circulation, 114(7), 700–752. URL http://dx.doi.org/10.1161/Circulationaha.106.177031

[7] Prystowsky, E. N., Benson, D. W., & Fuster, V. et al. (2000). Management of patients with atrial fibrillation: A statement for healthcare professionals from the subcommittee on electrocardiography and electrophysiology, American Heart Association. Circulation, 93 (6), 1262-1277. Retrieved August 9, 2011, from http://circ.ahajournals.org/content/93/6/1262.abstract

[8] Exception: It is rare, but an A-Fib patient may develop an extremely rapid, irregular heart rate which can be life threatening. It can strain your heart, reduce your circulation to dangerous levels, and make you feel like you're going to faint from lack of oxygen. In this situation, call the paramedics (dial 911 in the U.S.) or go to a hospital emergency room.

[9] Daccarett, M., Badger, T. J., Akoum, N., Burgon, N. S., et al. (2011). Association of left atrial fibrosis detected by Delayed-Enhancement magnetic resonance imaging and the risk of stroke in patients with atrial fibrillation. J Am Coll Cardiol , 57 (7), 831-838. URL http://dx.doi.org/10.1016/j.jacc.2010.09.049

[10] Gillinov, A. M., Blackstone, E. H., & McCarthy, P. M. (2002). Atrial fibrillation: current surgical options and their assessment. Ann Thorac Surg , 74 (6), 2210-2217. Retrieved September 3, 2011 from URL http://ats.ctsnetjournals.org/cgi/content/abstract/74/6/2210

[11] Blackshear, J. L., & Odell, J. A. (1985). Appendage obliteration to reduce stroke in cardiac surgical patients with atrial fibrillation. The Annals of thoracic surgery, 61 (2), 755-759. http://dx.doi.org/10.1016/0003-4975(95)00887-X

[12] Fuster, V., Rydén, L. E., Cannom, D. S. et al. (2006). ACC/AHA/ESC 2006 guidelines for the management of patients with atrial fibrillation—executive summary. Circulation, 114(7), 700–752. URL http://dx.doi.org/10.1161/Circulationaha.106.177031

[13] Abdon, N. J., Zettervall, O., Carlson, J. et al. (1982). Is occult atrial disorder a frequent cause of non-hemorrhagic stroke? Long-term ECG in 86 patients. Stroke, 13 (6), 832-837. Retrieved July 30, 2011, from http://stroke.ahajournals.org/content/13/6/832.abstract

[14] Schuchert, A., Behrens, G., & Meinertz, T. (1999). Impact of long-term ECG recording on the detection of paroxysmal atrial fibrillation in patients after an acute ischemic stroke. PACE, 22 (7), 1082-1084. Retrieved July 30, 2011, from http://view.ncbi.nlm.nih.gov/pubmed/10456638

[15] Furberg, C. (1994). Prevalence of atrial fibrillation in elderly subjects (the cardiovascular health study). The American Journal of Cardiology, 74 (3), 236-241. URL http://dx.doi.org/10.1016/0002-9149(94)90363-8

[16] Camm, A. J., Kirchhof, P., & Lip, G. Y. et al. (2010). Guidelines for the management of atrial fibrillation: The task force for the management of atrial fibrillation of the european society of cardiology (ESC). European Heart Journal, 31 (19), 2369-2429. URL http://dx.doi.org/10.1093/eurheartj/ehq278

[17] Loftus, B. D. (2002). Atrial fibrillation and stroke. Bellaire Neurology. Retrieved July 29, 2011, from http://www.loftusmd.com/Articles/stroke/atrialfibrillation.html

[18] Cardiovascular disease comprehensive 6–other connections: the link between infections and inflammation in heart disease. Life Extension Vitamins. Retrieved July 30, 2011, from http://www.lifeextensionvitamins.com/cadico6otco.html

[19] Fuster, V., Rydén, L. E., Cannom, D. S. et al. (2006). ACC/AHA/ESC 2006 guidelines for the management of patients with atrial fibrillation—executive summary. Circulation, 114(7), 700–752. URL http://dx.doi.org/10.1161/Circulationaha.106.177031

[20] Feinberg, W. M., Seeger, J. F., Carmody, R. F., et al. (1990). Epidemiologic features of asymptomatic cerebral infarction in patients with nonvalvular atrial fibrillation. Archives of internal medicine, 150 (11), 2340-2344. Retrieved September 11, 2011 from http://archinte.ama-assn.org/cgi/content/abstract/150/11/2340

[21] Veinot, J. P., Harrity, P. J., Gentile, F. et al. (1997). Anatomy of the normal left atrial appendage: A quantitative study of Age-Related changes in 500 autopsy hearts: Implications for echocardiographic examination. Circulation, 96 (9), 3112-3115. Retrieved September 11, 2011 from http://circ.ahajournals.org/content/96/9/3112.full

[22] Brown, M. T., & Bussell, J. K. (2011). Medication adherence: WHO cares? Mayo Clinic proceedings. Mayo Clinic , 86 (4), 304-314. URL http://dx.doi.org/10.4065/mcp.2010.0575

[23] ASA Plavix feasibility study with watchman left atrial appendage closure technology. ClinicalTrials.gov. Retrieved July 30, 2011, from http://clinicaltrials.gov/ct2/show/NCT00851578

[24] Evaluation of the Watchman LAA Closure Device in Patients With Atrial Fibrillation Versus Long Term Warfarin Therapy (PREVAIL) 2010. ClinicalTrials.gov. Retrieved July 30, 2011, from http://clinicaltrials.gov/ct2/show/NCT01182441?term=Watchman

[25] Bartus, K., Bednarek, J., & Myc, J. et al. (2010). Feasibility of closed-chest ligation of the left atrial appendage in Humans. Heart Rhythm, 8(2), 188-193. URL http://dx.doi.org/10.1016/j.hrthm.2010.10.040

[26] Peykar, S., & Estrada, J. C. (2010). Atrial fibrillation. Cardiac Arrhythmia Institute. Retrieved July 30, 2011, from http://www.caifl.com/atrial-fibrillation.html

[27] HeartScape: The chambers of the heart. 2005. SkillStat Learning. Retrieved July 30, 2011, from http://www.skillstat.com/heartscape/chambers.htm

[28] Feinberg, W. M., Seeger, J. F., Carmody, R. F., et al. (1990). Epidemiologic features of asymptomatic cerebral infarction in patients with nonvalvular atrial fibrillation. Archives of internal medicine, 150 (11), 2340-2344. Retrieved September 11, 2011 from http://archinte.ama-assn.org/cgi/content/abstract/150/11/2340

[29] Elias, M. F., Sullivan, L. M., Elias, P. K. et al. (2006). Atrial fibrillation is associated with lower cognitive performance in the framingham offspring men. Journal of stroke and cerebrovascular diseases, 15 (5), 214-222. URL http://dx.doi.org/10.1016/j.jstrokecerebrovasdis.2006.05.009

[30] Bunch, T. J., Weiss, J. P., Crandall, B. G., et al. (2010). Atrial fibrillation is independently associated with senile, vascular, and alzheimer's dementia. Heart Rhythm, 7 (4), 433-437. URL http://dx.doi.org/10.1016/j.hrthm.2009.12.004

[31] Peykar, S., & Estrada, J. C. Atrial fibrillation. Cardiac Arrhythmia Institute. Retrieved July 30, 2011, from http://www.caifl.com/atrial-fibrillation.html

[32] Bunch, T. J., Weiss, J. P., Crandall, B. G., et al. (2010). Atrial fibrillation is independently associated with senile, vascular, and alzheimer's dementia. Heart Rhythm, 7 (4), 433-437. URL http://dx.doi.org/10.1016/j.hrthm.2009.12.004

[33] Lloyd-Jones, D. M. (2004). Beyond the numbers: epidemiology and treatment of atrial fibrillation. Medscape Education. Retrieved July 30, 2011, from http://www.medscape.org/viewarticle/494006_2

[34] McCabe, P. J. (2010). Psychological distress in patients diagnosed with atrial fibrillation: the state of the science. The Journal of cardiovascular nursing, 25 (1), 40-51. URL http://dx.doi.org/10.1097/JCN.0b013e3181b7be36

[35] Lane, D. A., Langman, C. M., Lip, G. Y., & Nouwen, A. (2009). Illness perceptions, affective response, and health-related quality of life in patients with atrial fibrillation. Journal of psychosomatic research , 66 (3), 203-210. URL http://dx.doi.org/10.1016/j.jpsychores.2008.10.007

[36] O'Riordan, M. (2009). RECORD AF: Better success with rhythm control, but no difference in outcomes. Theheart.org. Retrieved August 01, 2011, from http://www.theheart.org/article/1023939.do

[37] ACC/AHA pocket guideline based on the ACC/AHA/ESC guidelines for the management of patients with atrial fibrillation management of patients with atrial fibrillation. July 2007. Retrieved July 30, 2011 from http://www.af-ablation.org/uploads/Management-of-Patients-with-atrial-fibrillation-pocket.pdf

[38] Wyndham, C. R. (2000). Atrial fibrillation: the most common arrhythmia. Texas Heart Institute journal /Texas Heart Institute of St. Luke's Episcopal Hospital, Texas Children's Hospital, 27 (3), 257-267. Retrieved August 9, 2011, from http://www.ncbi.nlm.nih.gov/pmc/articles/PMC101077/

[39] Schoonderwoerd, B. A., Smit, M. D., Pen, L. et al. (2008). New risk factors for atrial fibrillation: causes of 'not-so-lone atrial fibrillation'. Europace, 10 (6), 668-673. URL http://dx.doi.org/10.1093/europace/eun124

[40] Cardiovascular disease comprehensive 6–other connections: the link between infections and inflammation in heart disease. Life Extension Vitamins. Retrieved July 30, 2011, from http://www.lifeextensionvitamins.com/cadico6otco.html

[41] Villareal, R. P., Hariharan, R., Liu, B. C., et al. (2004). Postoperative atrial fibrillation and mortality after coronary artery bypass surgery. Journal of the American College of Cardiology , 43 (5), 742-748. URL http://dx.doi.org/10.1016/j.jacc.2003.11.023

[42] Maisel, W. H., Rawn, J. D., & Stevenson, W. G. (2001). Atrial fibrillation after cardiac surgery. Annals of internal medicine , 135 (12), 1061-1073. URL http://view.ncbi.nlm.nih.gov/pubmed/11747385

[43] Schoonderwoerd, B. A., Smit, M. D., Pen, L. et al. (2008). New risk factors for atrial fibrillation: causes of 'not-so-lone atrial fibrillation'. Europace, 10 (6), 668-673. URL http://dx.doi.org/10.1093/europace/eun124

[44] Heeringa, J., Kors, J. A., & Hofman, A. (2008). Cigarette smoking and risk of atrial fibrillation: the Rotterdam study. American heart journal , 156 (6), 1163-1169. URL http://dx.doi.org/10.1016/j.ahj.2008.08.003

[45] Sleep apnea and sleep. National Sleep Foundation. Retrieved July 30, 2011, from http://www.sleepfoundation.org/article/sleep-topics/sleep-apnea-and-sleep

[46] Calkins, H., & Berger, R. (2011) Johns Hopkins special reports: atrial fibrillation: the latest management strategies. p.11. ePub.

[47] Young, T., Palta, M., & Dempsey, J. (1993). The occurrence of sleep-disordered breathing among middle-aged adults. New England Journal of Medicine, 1993;328(17):1230-1235. Retrieved July 30, 2011 from http://www.nejm.org/doi/full/10.1056/NEJM199304293281704#t=abstract

[48] Ganz, L. I. (2011). Patient information: atrial fibrillation/atrial fibrillation causes. UpToDate Inc. Retrieved July 30, 2011 from http://www.uptodate.com/contents/patient-information-atrial-fibrillation#H

[49] Van Wagoner, D.R. (2005). Atrial selective strategies for treating atrial fibrillation. Drug Discovery Today: Therapeutic Strategies, 2(3): 291-295, 2005. Print. Abstract retrieved August 24, 2011 from http://pubget.com/paper/pgtmp_fe0042614504d62a4caa12c2a8d96415

[50] Go, A. S., Hylek, E. M., & Chang, Y. et al. (2001). Prevalence of diagnosed atrial fibrillation in adults: national implications for rhythm management and stroke prevention: the anticoagulation and risk factors in atrial fibrillation (ATRIA) study. Journal of the American Medical Association, 285(18), 2370-2375. URL http://dx.doi.org/10.1001/jama.285.18.2370

[51] Wolf, P. A., Abbott, R. D., & Kannel, W. B. (1987). Atrial fibrillation: a major contributor to stroke in the elderly. The framingham study. Archives of internal medicine, 147 (9), 1561-1564. Retrieved July 30, 2011 from URL http://view.ncbi.nlm.nih.gov/pubmed/3632164

[52] Feinberg, W. M., Blackshear, J. L., Laupacis, A., et al. (1995). Prevalence, age distribution, and gender of patients with atrial fibrillation. analysis and implications. Archives of internal medicine, 155 (5), 469-473. PubMed PMID: 7864703. Retrieved September 12, 2011 from http://www.ncbi.nlm.nih.gov/pubmed/7864703

[53] Van Wagoner, D.R. (2005). Atrial selective strategies for treating atrial fibrillation. Drug Discovery Today: Therapeutic Strategies, 2(3): 291-295, 2005. Print. Abstract retrieved August 24, 2011 from http://pubget.com/paper/pgtmp_fe0042614504d62a4caa12c2a8d96415

[54] Calkins, H., & Berger, R. (2011) Johns Hopkins special reports: atrial fibrillation: the latest management strategies. p.10. ePub.

[55] Kodama, S., Saito, K., & Tanaka, S. et al. (2011). Alcohol consumption and risk of atrial fibrillation: A Meta-Analysis. J Am Coll Cardiol , 57 (4), 427-436. Retrieved Nov. 19, 2011. URL http://dx.doi.org/10.1016/j.jacc.2010.08.641

[56] Lubitz, S. A., Yin, X., Fontes, J. D. et al. (2010). Association between familial atrial fibrillation and risk of new-onset atrial fibrillation. JAMA. 304 (20), 2263-2269. http://dx.doi.org/10.1001/jama.2010.1690

[57] Gonzalez, A. (July 07, 2011.). Atrial fibrillation is emerging as the new epidemic. Cardiac Rhythm News. Retrieved August 23, 2011, from http://www.cxvascular.com/crn-latest-

news/cardiac-rhythm-news---latest-news/atrial-fibrillation-is-emerging-as-the-new-epidemic

[58] Brugada, R., Tapscott, T., Czernuszewicz, G. Z. et al. (1997). Identification of a genetic locus for familial atrial fibrillation. New England Journal of Medicine, 336 (13), 905-911. http://dx.doi.org/10.1056/NEJM199703273361302

[59] Ludwig-Maximilians-Universität München. (2010).When the heart gets out of step: Newly identified gene may open route to innovative treatments for atrial fibrillation Press release. Retrieved July 30, 2011 from http://www.eurekalert.org/pub_releases/2010-02/lm-wth021910.php

[60] Mont, L., Elosua, R., & Brugada, J. (2009). Endurance sport practice as a risk factor for atrial fibrillation and atrial flutter. Europace, 11 (1), 11-17. URL http://dx.doi.org/10.1093/europace/eun289

[61] Karjalainen, J., Kujala, U. M., & Kaprio, J. et al. (1998). Lone atrial fibrillation in vigorously exercising middle aged men: case-control study. BMJ (Clinical research ed.), 316 (7147), 1784-1785. Retrieved August 01, 2011, from http://www.ncbi.nlm.nih.gov/pmc/articles/PMC28577/

[62] Metin, G., Yildiz, M., & Bayraktar, B. et al. (2010). Assessment of the P wave dispersion and duration in elite women basketball players. Indian Pacing Electrophysiol J. Retrieved August 01, 2011, from http://www.ncbi.nlm.nih.gov/pmc/articles/PMC2803602/

[63] Gonzalez, A. (July 07, 2011.). Atrial fibrillation is emerging as the new epidemic. Cardiac Rhythm News. Retrieved August 23, 2011, from http://www.cxvascular.com/crn-latest-news/cardiac-rhythm-news---latest-news/atrial-fibrillation-is-emerging-as-the-new-epidemic

[64] Wanahita, N., Messerli, F. H., Bangalore, S. et al. (2008). Atrial fibrillation and obesity-results of a meta-analysis. American heart journal, 155 (2), 310-315. URL http://dx.doi.org/10.1016/j.ahj.2007.10.004

[65] Women & Atrial Fibrillation. Center for Atrial Fibrillation, Northwestern Memorial Hospital. Retrieved July 31, 2011, from http://www.nmh.org/nm/women-and-atrial-fibrillation

[66] Who is at risk for atrial fibrillation? U.S. Department of Health & Human Services/National Institutes of Health. Retrieved August 1, 2011, from http://www.nhlbi.nih.gov/health/dci/Diseases/af/af_risk.html

[67] Cardiovascular disease comprehensive 6–other connections: the link between infections and inflammation in heart disease. Life Extension Vitamins. Retrieved July 30, 2011 from http://www.lifeextensionvitamins.com/cadico6otco.html

[68] Dell'Orfano, J. T., Luck, J. C., Wolbrette, D. L., Patel, H., & Naccarelli, G. V. (1998). Drugs for conversion of atrial fibrillation. American family physician , 58 (2), 471-480. Retrieved Nov. 19, 2011. URL http://view.ncbi.nlm.nih.gov/pubmed/9713400

[69] Kunz, J. S., Hemann, B., Edwin Atwood, J., et al. (2010). Is there a link between gastroesophageal reflux disease and atrial fibrillation? Clin Cardiol, 32 (10), 584-587. URL http://dx.doi.org/10.1002/clc.20660

[70] Barclay, L. (2005). Caffeine not associated with increased risk of atrial Fibrillation. Medscape News Today. Retrieved July 31, 2011, from http://www.medscape.com/viewarticle/501279?src=search%29

[71] Frost, L., & Vestergaard, P. (2005). Caffeine and risk of atrial fibrillation or flutter: the danish diet, cancer, and health study. The American Journal of Clinical Nutrition, 81 (3), 578-582. Retrieved July 30, 2011 from http://www.ajcn.org/content/81/3/578.abstract

[72] Katan, M. B., & Schouten, E. (2005). Caffeine and arrhythmia. The American Journal of Clinical Nutrition, 81 (3), 539-540. Retrieved July 30, 2011 from http://www.ajcn.org/content/81/3/539.abstract

[73] Ibid.

[74] Cohen, Todd J. A patient's guide to heart rhythm problems. Baltimore: Johns Hopkins UP, 2010. 171-72. Print.

[75] Cardiovascular disease comprehensive 8 - therapeutic C. Life Extension Vitamins. Retrieved July 30, 2011, from http://www.lifeextensionvitamins.com/cadico8thc.html

[76] Knox, K. (2008). An atrial fibrillation cause that you haven't been told.... Easy Immune System Health. Retrieved July 31, 2011, from http://www.easy-immune-health.com/atrial-fibrillation-cause.html

[77] Burgess, J. (2010). The strategy–what metabolic cardiology means to Afibbers. The AFIB Report, Hans R. Larsen, Editor. Retrieved July 30, 2011, from http://afibbers.org/resources/strategy.pdf

[78] Silver, B. B. (2004). Development of cellular magnesium nano-analysis in treatment of clinical magnesium deficiency. Journal of the American College of Nutrition, 23 (6), 732S-737S. Retrieved July 30, 2011, from http://www.jacn.org/content/23/6/732S.abstract

[79] McCarthy, J. T., & Kumar, R. Divalent Cation Metabolism: Magnesium, Chapter 4: *Disorders of Water, Electrolytes, and Acid-Base*, Vol. 1. R. W. Schrier (Ed.), 2000. The Atlas of Diseases of the Kidney series). Online chapter retrieved August 20, 2011 at http://www.cybernephrology.ualberta.ca/cn/Schrier/Volume1/chap4/ADK1_4_1-3.PDF

[80] Potassium online textbook. University of Tennessee Health Science Center, Division of Nephrology. Retrieved August 20, 2011 from http://www.uthsc.edu/nephrology/documents/potassium-textbook.pdf

[81] Potassium Supplements, *Vitamins & Health Supplements Guide*. (2005). Retrieved August 20, 2011, from http://www.vitamins-supplements.org/dietary-minerals/potassium.php

[82] The EXAtest measures intracellular levels of minerals such as magnesium, potassium and calcium. Accessed July 18, 2011 from http://www.exatest.com/

[83] Lazarides, L. Laboratory Tests for Nutritional Deficiencies. Health-Diets.Net: Nutrition Information and Resources from Linda Lazarides. Adapted from the Nutritional Health Bible by Linda Lazarides, 1998. Retrieved August 21, 2011, from http://www.health-diets.net/healthsearch/nutritionaldeftests.htm

[84] Woodard, MD, O. (2009, April 20). Magnesium: Do You Have Enough? *Great Health in Tough Times*. Retrieved August 21, 2011, from http://otiswoodardmd.typepad.com/my_weblog/2009/04/magnesium-do-you-have-enough.html

[85] Knox, K. (2008). An atrial fibrillation cause that you haven't been told.... Easy Immune System Health. Retrieved July 31, 2011, from http://www.easy-immune-health.com/atrial-fibrillation-cause.html

[86] King, D. E., Mainous, A. G., Geesey, M. E., et al. (2005). Dietary magnesium and c-reactive protein levels. Journal of the American College of Nutrition, 24 (3), 166-171. URL http://www.jacn.org/cgi/content/abstract/24/3/166

[87] Davis, W. (2007, February). Magnesium Deficiency: Is Your Bottled Water Killing You? Life Extension Magazine. Retrieved September 12, 2011, from http://www.lef.org/magazine/mag2007/feb2007_report_water_01.htm

[88] Stengler, M. (2011) Bottom Line Natural Healing. Vol.7, No.9, September 2011.

[89] Such as "Doctor's Best High Absorption 100% Chelated Magnesium."

[90] Such as "New Beginnings Liquid Magnesium-Ionic Liquid Concentrate."

[91] Understanding Arrhythmias: When the Beat Just Isn't Going on As Usual. Dr. Stephen Sinatra's Heart MD Institute,, P.A. Retrieved August 18, 2011 from http://www.heartmdinstitute.com/health-concerns/cardiovascular-system/heart-health/atrial-fibrillation-other-arrhythmias

[92] Seelig, M.S., and Rosanoff, A. The Magnesium Factor, 2003. p236.

[93] Sharma, K. (2011). Calcium to magnesium ratio. Enerex Botanicals Ltd. Retrieved July 31, 2011 from http://www.enerex.ca/en/articles/calcium-to-magnesium-ratio

[94] Stengler, M. (2011) Bottom Line Natural Healing. Vol.7, No.9, September 2011.

[95] Knox, K. (2008). An atrial fibrillation cause that you haven't been told... Easy Immune System Health. Retrieved July 31, 2011, from http://www.easy-immune-health.com/atrial-fibrillation-cause.html

[96] One source of magnesium oil is "Ancient Minerals Ultra-Pure Magnesium" which is odorless.

[97] Natale, A., & Jalife, J. Atrial fibrillation from bench to bedside. Totowa, NJ: Humana Press. 2008. 103-104. Print.

[98] Sharma, K. (2011). Calcium to magnesium ratio. Enerex Botanicals Ltd. Retrieved July 31, 2011 from http://www.enerex.ca/en/articles/calcium-to-magnesium-ratio

[99] Dean, Carol. The Magnesium Miracle. 2007. Ballantine Books.

[100] Dietary Reference Intakes for Calcium and Vitamin D: Report Brief. Revised March 2011, Institute of Medicine of the National Academies. Retrieved August 31, 2011. URL http://www.iom.edu/Reports/2010/Dietary-Reference-Intakes-for-Calcium-and-Vitamin-D.aspx

[101] Berkelhammer, C., & Bear, R. A. (1985). A clinical approach to common electrolyte problems: 4. hypomagnesemia. Canadian Medical Association journal, 132 (4), 360-368. Retrieved July 31, 2011 from http://www.ncbi.nlm.nih.gov/pmc/articles/PMC1345822/

[102] Electrolyte Imbalance - Normal Adult Values. 2005. Chemo Care. Content provided by Cleveland Clinic Cancer Center. Retrieved August 19, 2011, from http://www.chemocare.com/managing/electrolyte_imbalance.asp

[103] EXAtest sample report; Retrieved August 16, 2011 from http://www.exatest.com/PDF%20Files/report1.jpg

[104] Seelig, M.S., and Rosanoff, A. The Magnesium Factor, 2003. p236.

[105] Appel, L. J. (chair). (2004). Dietary reference intakes for water, potassium, sodium, chloride, and sulfate. Consensus report. Panel on dietary reference intakes for electrolytes and water. The National Academies Press. Retrieved July 31, 2011, from http://books.nap.edu/openbook.php?record_id=10925

[106] Van Wagoner, D. R. (2003). Atrial fibrillation and potassium. Common questions and answers/resources for patients/Cleveland Clinic. Retrieved July 31, 2011 from http://my.clevelandclinic.org/heart/askdoctor/afib_potassium.aspx

[107] Understanding Arrhythmias: When the Beat Just Isn't Going on As Usual. Dr. Stephen Sinatra's Heart MD Institute,, P.A. Retrieved August 18, 2011 from http://www.heartmdinstitute.com/health-concerns/cardiovascular-system/heart-health/atrial-fibrillation-other-arrhythmias

[108] Such as "NOW Potassium Gluconate Powder-1 lb. container.

[109] Knox, K. (2008). An atrial fibrillation cause that you haven't been told.... Easy Immune System Health. Retrieved July 31, 2011, from http://www.easy-immune-health.com/atrial-fibrillation-cause.html

[110] Ibid

[110] Van Wagoner, D. R. (2003). Atrial fibrillation and potassium. Common questions and answers/resources for patients/Cleveland Clinic. Retrieved July 31, 2011 from http://my.clevelandclinic.org/heart/askdoctor/afib_potassium.aspx

[111] Recommended Dietary Allowances (RDA): the daily dietary intake level of a nutrient considered sufficient by the Food and Nutrition Board to meet the requirements of nearly all (97–98%) healthy individuals in each life-stage and gender group; Adequate Intake (AI): where no RDA has been established, but the amount established is somewhat less firmly believed to be adequate for everyone in the demographic group.

Both are part of the Dietary Reference Intake (DRI) system of nutrition recommendations from the Institute of Medicine (IOM) of the U.S. National Academy of Sciences; Retrieved August 16, 2011 from http://www.cnpp.usda.gov/Publications/DietaryGuidelines/2010/PolicyDoc/Appendices.pdf

[112] Seelig, M.S., and Rosanoff, A. The Magnesium Factor, 2003. p236.

[113] Understanding Arrhythmias: When the Beat Just Isn't Going on As Usual. Dr. Stephen Sinatra's Heart MD Institute,, P.A. Retrieved August 18, 2011 from http://www.heartmdinstitute.com/health-concerns/cardiovascular-system/heart-health/atrial-fibrillation-other-arrhythmias

[114] NOW Foods - Potassium Gluconate Powder - 1 lb. NOW Foods. Retrieved August 19, 2011, from http://www.nowfoods.com/Products/M095343.htm

[115] Cardiovascular disease comprehensive 8 - therapeutic C. Life Extension Vitamins. Retrieved July 30, 2011, from http://www.lifeextensionvitamins.com/cadico8thc.html

[116] Knox, K. (2008). An atrial fibrillation cause that you haven't been told.... Easy Immune System Health. Retrieved July 31, 2011, from http://www.easy-immune-health.com/atrial-fibrillation-cause.html

[117] Sinatra, S. T. (2011). Understanding arrhythmias/causes of arrhythmia/electrolyte imbalances. Heart MD Institute. Retrieved August 1, 2011, from http://www.heartmdinstitute.com/health-concerns/cardiovascular-system/heart-health/atrial-fibrillation-other-arrhythmias

[118] Ibid.

[119] Berkelhammer, C., & Bear, R. A. (1985). A clinical approach to common electrolyte problems: 4. hypomagnesemia. Canadian Medical Association journal, 132 (4), 360-368. Retrieved July 31, 2011 from http://www.ncbi.nlm.nih.gov/pmc/articles/PMC1345822/

[120] Natale, A., & Jalife, J. Atrial fibrillation from bench to bedside. Totowa, NJ: Humana Press. 2008. 103-104. Print.

[121] Wyse, D. G. (1997). Atrial fibrillation: the clinically relevant trials and results. Annual Scientific Session of the American College of Cardiology, Anaheim, California. (1997, March). Retrieved July 31, 2011, from http://www.pslgroup.com/dg/25f9a.htm

[122] Maugh, II, T. H. (2010, November 16). New drugs may replace problematic blood thinner. Los Angeles Times, p.A12.

[123] Pradaxa. Boehringer Ingelheim Pharmaceuticals Inc. (2010). Full Prescribing Information, Clinical Trials Experience, Gastrointestinal Adverse Reactions. Retrieved July 31, 2011, from http://dailymed.nlm.nih.gov/dailymed/lookup.cfm?setid=ba74e3cd-b06f-4145-b284-5fd6b84ff3c9

[124] Ibid.

[125] Haines, D. E. Atrial fibrillation: new approaches in management, presented by Dr. David Haines. (1999, August 10). [Transcript, Television broadcast]. University of Virginia School of Medicine. Retrieved July 31, 2011 from http://www.a-fib.com/HainesUnOfVirginiaAtrialFibrillation.htm

[126] ASA Plavix feasibility study with watchman left atrial appendage closure technology. ClinicalTrials.gov. Retrieved July 30, 2011, from http://clinicaltrials.gov/ct2/show/NCT00851578

[127] Evaluation of the Watchman LAA Closure Device in Patients With Atrial Fibrillation Versus Long Term Warfarin Therapy (PREVAIL) 2010. ClinicalTrials.gov. Retrieved July 30, 2011, from http://clinicaltrials.gov/ct2/show/NCT01182441?term=Watchman

[128] Bartus, K., Bednarek, J., & Myc, J. et al. (2010). Feasibility of closed-chest ligation of the left atrial appendage in Humans. Heart Rhythm, 8(2), 188-193. URL http://dx.doi.org/10.1016/j.hrthm.2010.10.040

[129] Drug treatment for atrial fibrillation. 2011. The London Atrial Fibrillation Centre. Retrieved July 31, 2011, from http://www.londonafcentre.co.uk/atrial_fibrillation_treatmentdrugs_for_af

[130] Ibid

[131] Haines, D. E. Atrial fibrillation: new approaches in management, presented by Dr. David Haines. (1999, August 10). [Transcript, Television broadcast]. University of Virginia School of Medicine. Retrieved July 31, 2011 from http://www.a-fib.com/HainesUnOfVirginiaAtrialFibrillation.htm

[132] Ibid

[133] O'Riordan, M. (2009). RECORD AF: Better success with rhythm control, but no difference in outcomes. Theheart.org. Retrieved August 01, 2011, from http://www.theheart.org/article/1023939.do

[134] Sotalol has characteristics of both a Class II [Beta Blocker] and Class III drug.

[135] Amiodarone has characteristics of both Class I and Class III drugs.

[136] Dronedarone (Multaq) has characteristics of both Class I and Class III drugs.

[137] Cannom, D. S. (2000). Atrial fibrillation: nonpharmacologic approaches. American Journal of Cardiology, 85(10), 1, 25-35. Retrieved July 31, 2011 from http://www.ajconline.org/article/S0002-9149(00)00904-8/abstract

[138] Haines, D. E. Atrial fibrillation: new approaches in management, presented by Dr. David Haines. (1999, August 10). [Transcript, Television broadcast]. University of Virginia School of Medicine. Retrieved July 31, 2011 from http://www.a-fib.com/HainesUnOfVirginiaAtrialFibrillation.htm

[139] Falk, R. H. (2001). Atrial fibrillation. New England Journal of Medicine, 344 (14), 1067-1078. URL http://dx.doi.org/10.1056/NEJM200104053441407

[140] Siddoway, L. A. (2003). Amiodarone: guidelines for use and monitoring. American family physician, 68 (11), 2189-2196. Retrieved Nov. 19, 2011. URL http://view.ncbi.nlm.nih.gov/pubmed/14677664

[141] Medifocus guidebook on: atrial fibrillation: a comprehensive guide to symptoms, treatment, research, and support. Medifocus.com, Inc. July 2010. Vol. #CR004. 40. Print.

[142] Savelieva I, Camm J. Update on atrial fibrillation: part II. Clin Cardiol. 2008 Mar;31(3):102-8. Review. PubMed PMID: 18383050. URL Retrieved Nov 17, 2011. http://www.ncbi.nlm.nih.gov/pubmed?term=PMID%3A%2018383050

[143] Wyndham, C. R. (2000). Atrial fibrillation: the most common arrhythmia. Texas Heart Institute journal /Texas Heart Institute of St. Luke's Episcopal Hospital, Texas Children's Hospital, 27 (3), 257-267. Retrieved August 9, 2011, from http://www.ncbi.nlm.nih.gov/pmc/articles/PMC101077/

[144] Gupta, D. Atrial fibrillation: which treatment strategy? Ablation or drugs? HeartRhythmSpecialist.co.uk. Retrieved July 31, 2011, from http://www.heartrhythmspecialist.co.uk/Heartrhythmspecialist.co.uk/AF__Ablation_or_drugs.html

[145] Haines, D. E. Atrial fibrillation: new approaches in management, presented by Dr. David Haines. (1999, August 10). [Transcript, Television broadcast]. University of Virginia School of Medicine. Retrieved July 31, 2011 from http://www.a-fib.com/HainesUnOfVirginiaAtrialFibrillation.htm

[146] Fuster, V., Rydén, L. E., Cannom, D. S. et al. (2006). ACC/AHA/ESC 2006 guidelines for the management of patients with atrial fibrillation—executive summary. Circulation, 114(7), 700–752. URL http://dx.doi.org/10.1161/Circulationaha.106.177031

[147] Atrial Fibrillation. InteliHealth: (2008). Medical content reviewed by the faulty of Harvard Medical School. Retrieved July 31, 2011, from http://www.intelihealth.com/IH/ihtIH/WSIHW000/9339/23923.html

[148] Jaïs, P., Weerasooriya, R., Shah, D. C. et al. (2002). Ablation therapy for atrial fibrillation (AF): past, present and future. Cardiovascular Research, 54 (2), 337-346. URL http://dx.doi.org/10.1016/S0008-6363(02)00263-8

[149] Haïssaguerre, M., Jaïs, P., Shah, D. C. et al. (1998). Spontaneous initiation of atrial fibrillation by ectopic beats originating in the pulmonary veins. The New England journal of medicine, 339 (10), 659-666. URL http://dx.doi.org/10.1056/NEJM199809033391003

[150] Radiofrequency catheter ablation is considered safe. (2010). AFIB Alliance: Atrial Fibrillation Resource. Retrieved August 01, 2011, from http://www.atrialfibrillation.com/medical-prof/therapy-outcome/safety

[151] Answering your questions about the electrophysiology study. St. Paul, MN: Boston Scientific, 2008. Cardiac Rhythm Management. C1-196-0808. p 10. Retrieved July 31, 2011, from http://www.bostonscientific.com/lifebeat-online/assets/pdfs/resources/C1-196_0808_EPSPatientBroch.pdf

[152] Fuster, V., Rydén, L. E., Cannom, D. S. et al. (2006). ACC/AHA/ESC 2006 guidelines for the management of patients with atrial fibrillation—executive summary. Circulation, 114(7), 700–752. URL http://dx.doi.org/10.1161/Circulationaha.106.177031

[153] Lin, W.-S. S., Tai, C.-T. T., & Hsieh, M.-H. H. et al. (2003). Catheter ablation of paroxysmal atrial fibrillation initiated by non-pulmonary vein ectopy. Circulation , 107 (25), 3176-3183. URL http://dx.doi.org/10.1161/01.CIR.0000074206.52056.2D

[154] Ciaccio, E. J., Biviano, A. B., Whang, W. et al. (2010). Different characteristics of complex fractionated atrial electrograms in acute paroxysmal versus long-standing persistent atrial fibrillation. Heart rhythm, 7 (9), 1207-1215. URL http://dx.doi.org/10.1016/j.hrthm.2010.06.018

[155] Nainggolan, L. (2008). Cryoablation: Safer than RF but slightly lower success rate? Theheart.org by WebMD. Retrieved August 1, 2011, from http://www.theheart.org/article/877315.do

[156] Kühne, M., Schaer, B., Ammann, P., et al. (2010). Cryoballoon ablation for pulmonary vein isolation in patients with paroxysmal atrial fibrillation. Swiss Med Wkly. 2010 Apr 17;140 (15-16), 214-221. Abstract. PubMed PMID:20407957

[157] Marijon, E., Albenque, J.-P. P., & Boveda, S. (2009). Feasibility and safety of same-day home discharge after radiofrequency catheter ablation. The American journal of cardiology , 104 (2), 254-258. URL http://dx.doi.org/10.1016/j.amjcard.2009.03.024

[158] Cappato, R., Calkins, H., & Chen, S.-A. (2010). Updated worldwide survey on the methods, efficacy, and safety of catheter ablation for human atrial fibrillation / CLINICAL PERSPECTIVE. Circulation: Arrhythmia and Electrophysiology, 3 (1), 32-38. URL http://dx.doi.org/10.1161/CIRCEP.109.859116

[159] Haïssaguerre, M., Jaïs, P., Shah, D. C. et al. (2000). Electrophysiological end point for catheter ablation of atrial fibrillation initiated from multiple pulmonary venous foci. Circulation, 101 (12), 1409-1417. Retrieved August 01, 2011, from http://view.ncbi.nlm.nih.gov/pubmed/10736285

[160] Jaïs, P., Weerasooriya, R., Shah, D. C. et al. (2002). Ablation therapy for atrial fibrillation (AF): past, present and future. Cardiovascular Research, 54 (2), 337-346. URL http://dx.doi.org/10.1016/S0008-6363(02)00263-8

[161] Jais, P. Improved A-Fib Procedure. Summary of peer presentation. North American Society of Pacing and Electrophysiology Convention (NASPE), San Diego, CA May, 2002, San Diego. Retrieved July 31, 2011 from http://www.a-fib.com/HeartRhythmSociety2002.htm

[162] Cappato, R., Calkins, H., & Chen, S.-A. (2010). Updated worldwide survey on the methods, efficacy, and safety of catheter ablation for human atrial fibrillation / CLINICAL PERSPECTIVE. Circulation: Arrhythmia and Electrophysiology, 3 (1), 32-38. URL http://dx.doi.org/10.1161/CIRCEP.109.859116

[163] Kuck, K. H. Five-year follow-up of catheter ablation for PAF. Summary of peer presentation. Boston Atrial Fibrillation Symposium, Boston, MA. January, 14, 2011. Retrieved July 31, 2011 from http://www.a-fib.com/BostonA-FibSymposium2011.htm

[164] Ouyang, F., Tilz, R., & Chun, J. (2010). Long-Term results of catheter ablation in paroxysmal atrial fibrillation: Lessons from a 5-Year Follow-Up. Circulation, 122 (23), 2368-2377. URL http://dx.doi.org/10.1161/Circulationaha.110.946806

[165] Marchlinski, F. Pulmonary Vein Isolation Alone for Long Standing Persistent A-Fib. Summary of peer presentation. Boston Atrial Fibrillation Symposium, Boston, MA. January, 14, 2011. Retrieved July 31, 2011 from http://www.a-fib.com/BostonA-FibSymposium2011.htm

[166] Wilber, D. (2011). Very late recurrence after catheter ablation of AF: Incidence and implications. Summary of peer presentation. Boston Atrial Fibrillation Symposium, Boston, MA. January, 14, 2011. Retrieved July 31, 2011 from http://www.a-fib.com/BostonA-FibSymposium2011.htm

[167] O'Riordan, M. (2011, January 5). Sobering long-term outcomes following ablation of atrial fibrillation. Theheart.org. Retrieved August 01, 2011, from http://www.theheart.org/article/1168671.do

[168] Sawhney, N., Anousheh, R., Chen, W.-C. C. et al. (2009). Five-year outcomes after segmental pulmonary vein isolation for paroxysmal atrial fibrillation. The American journal of cardiology, 104 (3), 366-372. URL http://dx.doi.org/10.1016/j.amjcard.2009.03.044

[169] Bunch, J. J., Crandall, B. G., & Weiss, P. P. (2011). Patients treated with catheter ablation for atrial fibrillation have long-term rates of death, stroke, and dementia similar to patients without atrial fibrillation. Journal of cardiovascular electrophysiology , 22 (8), 839-845. URL http://dx.doi.org/10.1111/j.1540-8167.2011.02035.x

[170] Jais, P. Improved A-Fib Procedure. Summary of peer presentation. North American Society of Pacing and Electrophysiology Convention (NASPE), San Diego, CA May, 2002, San Diego. Retrieved July 31, 2011 from http://www.a-fib.com/HeartRhythmSociety2002.htm

[171] Calkins, H., Brugada, J., & Packer, D. L. et al. (2007). HRS/EHRA/ECAS expert Consensus Statement on catheter and surgical ablation of atrial fibrillation: recommendations for personnel, policy, procedures and follow-up. A report of the Heart Rhythm Society (HRS) Task Force on catheter and surgical ablation of atrial fibrillation. VII Outcomes and efficacy of catheter ablation of atrial fibrillation. Europace, 9, 335-379. URL http://dx.doi.org/10.1093/europace/eun341

[172] Nainggolan, L. (2008). Cryoablation: Safer than RF but slightly lower success rate? Theheart.org by WebMD. Retrieved August 1, 2011, from http://www.theheart.org/article/877315.do

[173] Savelieva, I., & Camm, A. J. (2000). Clinical relevance of silent atrial fibrillation: prevalence, prognosis, quality of life, and management. Journal of interventional cardiac, 4 (2), 369-382. Retrieved July 31, 2011 from http://view.ncbi.nlm.nih.gov/pubmed/10936003

[174] Elias, M. F., Sullivan, L. M., Elias, P. K. et al. (2006). Atrial fibrillation is associated with lower cognitive performance in the framingham offspring men. Journal of stroke and cerebrovascular diseases, 15 (5), 214-222. URL http://dx.doi.org/10.1016/j.jstrokecerebrovasdis.2006.05.009

[175] Scheinman, M. M., & Morady, F. (2001). Nonpharmacological approaches to atrial fibrillation. Circulation, 103 (16), 2120-2125. Retrieved July 31, 2011 from http://circ.ahajournals.org/content/103/16/2120.abstract

[176] Damiano, R. J., Gaynor, S. L., Bailey, M. et al. (2003). The long-term outcome of patients with coronary disease and atrial fibrillation undergoing the Cox-Maze procedure. The

Journal of thoracic and cardiovascular surgery, 126 (6), 2016-2021. URL
http://dx.doi.org/10.1016/j.jtcvs.2003.07.006

[177] Ibid.

[178] Medifocus guidebook on: atrial fibrillation: a comprehensive guide to symptoms,
treatment, research, and support. Medifocus.com, Inc. July 2010. Vol. #CR004. 40. Print.

[179] Lall, S. C., Melby, S. J., Voeller, R. K. et al. (2007). The effect of ablation technology on
surgical outcomes after the Cox-Maze procedure: A propensity analysis. J Thorac
Cardiovasc Surg, 133 (2), 389-396. URL http://dx.doi.org/10.1016/j.jtcvs.2006.10.009

[180] Damiano, R. J. (2008, February 15). The Cox-Maze IV Procedure: Operative Technique and
Results. Slide set. Presented at First Crossing Borders AF Meeting in Netherlands,
Maastricht. Retrieved August 22, 2011 from http://www.crossing-
borders.info/presentaties/damiano.pdf

[181] Damiano, R. J., & Bailey, M. (2007). The Cox-Maze IV procedure for lone atrial fibrillation.
MMCTS , 2007 (0723), 2758+. URL http://dx.doi.org/10.1510/mmcts.2007.002758

[182] Medifocus guidebook on: atrial fibrillation: a comprehensive guide to symptoms,
treatment, research, and support. Medifocus.com, Inc. July 2010. Vol. #CR004. 40. Print.

[183] Damiano, R. J. (2008). What is the best way to surgically eliminate the left atrial
appendage? Journal of the American College of Cardiology, 52 (11), 930-931. URL
http://dx.doi.org/10.1016/j.jacc.2008.06.007

[184] Narumiya, T. et al. "Relationship between left atrial appendage function and left atrial
thrombus in patients with nonvalvular chronic atrial fibrillation and atrial flutter." Circ. J
2003 Jan;67(1):68-72. URL http://www.ncbi.nlm.nih.gov/pubmed/12520155

[185] Edgerton, J. R., McClelland, J. H., Duke, D. et al. (2009). Minimally invasive surgical ablation
of atrial fibrillation: six-month results. The Journal of thoracic and cardiovascular
surgery, 138 (1). URL http://dx.doi.org/10.1016/j.jtcvs.2008.09.080

[186] Han, F. T., Kasirajan, V., Kowalski, M., et al. (2009). Results of a minimally invasive surgical
pulmonary vein isolation and ganglionic plexi ablation for atrial fibrillation: single-center
experience with 12-month follow-up. Circulation. Arrhythmia and electrophysiology, 2
(4), 370-377. URL http://dx.doi.org/10.1161/CIRCEP.109.854828

[187] Wolf, R. K., Schneeberger, E. W., Osterday, R., Miller, D. et al. (2005). Video-assisted
bilateral pulmonary vein isolation and left atrial appendage exclusion for atrial
fibrillation. The Journal of thoracic and cardiovascular surgery, 130 (3), 797-802. URL
http://dx.doi.org/10.1016/j.jtcvs.2005.03.041

[188] Minimally-invasive radiofrequency ablation for atrial fibrillation. Johns Hopkins Medicine.
Retrieved August 01, 2011, from
http://www.hopkinsmedicine.org/heart_vascular_institute/conditions_treatments/treat
ments/minimally_invasive_radiofrequency_ablation.html

[189] Han, F. T., Kasirajan, V., Kowalski, M., et al. (2009). Results of a minimally invasive surgical
pulmonary vein isolation and ganglionic plexi ablation for atrial fibrillation: single-center
experience with 12-month follow-up. Circulation. Arrhythmia and electrophysiology, 2
(4), 370-377. URL http://dx.doi.org/10.1161/CIRCEP.109.854828

[190] Kron, J., Kasirajan, V., Wood, M. A., et al. (2010). Management of recurrent atrial
arrhythmias after minimally invasive surgical pulmonary vein isolation and ganglionic
plexi ablation for atrial fibrillation. Heart rhythm, 7 (4), 445-451. URL
http://dx.doi.org/10.1016/j.hrthm.2009.12.008

[191] Atrial Fibrillation Health Center: Pacemaker for atrial fibrillation. (2010, November 2).
WebMD. Retrieved August 28, 2011, from http://www.webmd.com/heart-disease/atrial-
fibrillation/pacemaker-for-atrial-fibrillation

[192] Yamada, T., Murakami, Y., Okada, T. et al. (2008). Electroanatomic mapping in the catheter ablation of premature atrial contractions with a non-pulmonary vein origin. Europace, 10 (11), 1320-1324. URL http://dx.doi.org/10.1093/europace/eun238

[193] O'Riordan, M. (2009). RECORD AF: Better success with rhythm control, but no difference in outcomes. Theheart.org. Retrieved August 01, 2011, from http://www.theheart.org/article/1023939.do

[194] Haïssaguerre, M., Jaïs, P., Shah, D. C. et al. (2000). Electrophysiological end point for catheter ablation of atrial fibrillation initiated from multiple pulmonary venous foci. Circulation, 101 (12), 1409-1417. Retrieved August 01, 2011, from http://view.ncbi.nlm.nih.gov/pubmed/10736285

[195] Jais, P. Improved A-Fib Procedure. Summary of peer presentation. North American Society of Pacing and Electrophysiology Convention (NASPE), San Diego, CA May, 2002, San Diego. Retrieved July 31, 2011 from http://www.a-fib.com/HeartRhythmSociety2002.htm

[196] Navarrete, A., Conte, F., Moran, M., Ali, I., & Milikan, N. (2011). Ablation of atrial fibrillation at the time of cavotricuspid isthmus ablation in patients with atrial flutter without documented atrial fibrillation derives a better Long-Term benefit. Journal of Cardiovascular Electrophysiology , 22 (1), 34-38. URL http://dx.doi.org/10.1111/j.1540-8167.2010.01845.x

[197] Ibid.

[198] Ibid.

[199] Katkhouda, N., Mason, R. J., Towfigh, S., et al. (2005). Laparoscopic versus open appendectomy: a prospective randomized double-blind study. Annals of surgery, 242 (3). Retrieved Nov 30, 2011. URL http://www.ncbi.nlm.nih.gov/pmc/articles/PMC1357752/

[200] Radiofrequency catheter ablation is considered safe. (2010). AFIB Alliance: Atrial Fibrillation Resource. Retrieved August 01, 2011, from http://www.atrialfibrillation.com/medical-prof/therapy-outcome/safety

[201] Professional answers to your atrial fibrillation questions: what are the risks of AF ablation? Atrial Fibrillation Institute/St. Vincent's HealthCare. Retrieved August 01, 2011, from http://www.afibjax.com/faq.php

[202] Ibid.

[203] Jaïs, P., Weerasooriya, R., Shah, D. C. et al. (2002). Ablation therapy for atrial fibrillation (AF): past, present and future. Cardiovascular Research, 54 (2), 337-346. URL http://dx.doi.org/10.1016/S0008-6363(02)00263-8

[204] Bucerius, J., Gummert, J. F., Borger, M. A., et al. (2003). Stroke after cardiac surgery: a risk factor analysis of 16,184 consecutive adult patients. Ann Thorac Surg, 75 (2), 472-478. Retrieved July 30, 2011, from http://ats.ctsnetjournals.org/cgi/content/abstract/75/2/472

[205] Open Heart Surgery Complications. (2006, November 1). EMedTV. Retrieved September 17, 2011, from http://heart-disease.emedtv.com/open-heart-surgery/open-heart-surgery-complications-p2.html

[206] Ibid.

[207] Schaff, H. V., Dearani, J. A., Daly, R. C., et al. (2000). Cox-Maze procedure for atrial fibrillation: Mayo clinic experience. Seminars in thoracic and cardiovascular surgery, 12 (1), 30-37. Retrieved September 14, 2011, from http://view.ncbi.nlm.nih.gov/pubmed/10746920

[208] Mueller, D. K. (2009, June 4). Mediastinitis: Overview/Background. *Medscape Reference.* Retrieved September 17, 2011, from http://emedicine.medscape.com/article/425308-overview

[209] Schaff, H. V., Dearani, J. A., Daly, R. C., et al. (2000). Cox-Maze procedure for atrial fibrillation: Mayo clinic experience. Seminars in thoracic and cardiovascular surgery, 12

(1), 30-37. Retrieved September 14, 2011, from
http://view.ncbi.nlm.nih.gov/pubmed/10746920

[210] Marchlinski, F. Pulmonary Vein Isolation Alone for Long Standing Persistent A-Fib.
Summary of peer presentation. Boston Atrial Fibrillation Symposium, Boston, MA.
January, 14, 2011. Retrieved July 31, 2011 from http://www.a-
fib.com/BostonA-FibSymposium2011.htm

[211] Wilber, D. (2011). Very late recurrence after catheter ablation of AF: Incidence and
implications. Summary of peer presentation. Boston Atrial Fibrillation Symposium,
Boston, MA. January, 14, 2011. Retrieved July 31, 2011 from http://www.a-
fib.com/BostonA-FibSymposium2011.htm

[212] O'Riordan, M. (2011, January 5). Sobering long-term outcomes following ablation of atrial
fibrillation. Theheart.org. Retrieved August 01, 2011, from
http://www.theheart.org/article/1168671.do

[213] Sawhney, N., Anousheh, R., Chen, W.-C. C. et al. (2009). Five-year outcomes after
segmental pulmonary vein isolation for paroxysmal atrial fibrillation. The American
journal of cardiology, 104 (3), 366-372. URL
http://dx.doi.org/10.1016/j.amjcard.2009.03.044

[214] Damiano, R. J. (2008, February 15). The Cox-Maze IV Procedure: Operative Technique and
Results. Slide set. Presented at First Crossing Borders AF Meeting in Netherlands,
Maastricht. Retrieved August 22, 2011 from http://www.crossing-
borders.info/presentaties/damiano.pdf

[215] Han, F. T., Kasirajan, V., Kowalski, M., et al. (2009). Results of a minimally invasive surgical
pulmonary vein isolation and ganglionic plexi ablation for atrial fibrillation: single-center
experience with 12-month follow-up. Circulation. Arrhythmia and electrophysiology, 2
(4), 370-377. URL http://dx.doi.org/10.1161/CIRCEP.109.854828

[216] Kron, J., Kasirajan, V., Wood, M. A., et al. (2010). Management of recurrent atrial
arrhythmias after minimally invasive surgical pulmonary vein isolation and ganglionic
plexi ablation for atrial fibrillation. Heart rhythm, 7 (4), 445-451. URL
http://dx.doi.org/10.1016/j.hrthm.2009.12.008

[217] Wyndham, C. R. (2000). Atrial fibrillation: the most common arrhythmia. Texas Heart
Institute journal /Texas Heart Institute of St. Luke's Episcopal Hospital, Texas Children's
Hospital, 27 (3), 257-267. Retrieved August 9, 2011, from
http://www.ncbi.nlm.nih.gov/pmc/articles/PMC101077/

[218] Jais, P. Improved A-Fib Procedure. Summary of peer presentation. North American Society
of Pacing and Electrophysiology Convention (NASPE), San Diego, CA May, 2002, San
Diego. Retrieved July 31, 2011 from http://www.a-fib.com/HeartRhythmSociety2002.htm

[219] Calkins, H., Brugada, J., & Packer, D. L. et al. (2007). HRS/EHRA/ECAS expert Consensus
Statement on catheter and surgical ablation of atrial fibrillation: recommendations for
personnel, policy, procedures and follow-up. A report of the Heart Rhythm Society
(HRS) Task Force on catheter and surgical ablation of atrial fibrillation. VII Outcomes
and efficacy of catheter ablation of atrial fibrillation. Europace, 9, 335-379. URL
http://dx.doi.org/10.1093/europace/eun341

[220] Atrial Fibrillation. InteliHealth: (2008). Medical content reviewed by the faulty of Harvard
Medical School. Retrieved July 31, 2011, from
http://www.intelihealth.com/IH/ihtIH/WSIHW000/9339/23923.html

[221] Savelieva, I., & Camm, A. J. (2000). Clinical relevance of silent atrial fibrillation: prevalence,
prognosis, quality of life, and management. Journal of interventional cardiac, 4 (2), 369-
382. Retrieved July 31, 2011 from http://view.ncbi.nlm.nih.gov/pubmed/10936003

[222] Atrial Fibrillation. InteliHealth: (2008). Medical content reviewed by the faulty of Harvard Medical School. Retrieved July 31, 2011, from http://www.intelihealth.com/IH/ihtIH/WSIHW000/9339/23923.html

[223] Haines, D. E. Atrial fibrillation: new approaches in management, presented by Dr. David Haines. (1999, August 10). [Transcript, Television broadcast]. University of Virginia School of Medicine. Retrieved July 31, 2011 from http://www.a-fib.com/HainesUnOfVirginiaAtrialFibrillation.htm

[224] Haïssaguerre, M., Hocini, M., & Sanders, P. (2005). Catheter ablation of long-lasting persistent atrial fibrillation: clinical outcome and mechanisms of subsequent arrhythmias. Journal of cardiovascular electrophysiology, 16 (11), 1138-1147. URL http://dx.doi.org/10.1111/j.1540-8167.2005.00308.x

[225] Romano, M. A., Bach, D. S., & Pagani, F. D. (2004). Atrial reduction plasty Cox-Maze procedure: extended indications for atrial fibrillation surgery. The Annals of thoracic surgery, 77 (4). URL http://dx.doi.org/10.1016/j.athoracsur.2003.06.022

[226] Damiano, R. J. (2008). What is the best way to surgically eliminate the left atrial appendage? Journal of the American College of Cardiology, 52 (11), 930-931. URL http://dx.doi.org/10.1016/j.jacc.2008.06.007

[227] Cappato, R., Calkins, H., & Chen, S.-A. et al. Updated worldwide survey on the methods, efficacy, and safety of catheter ablation for human atrial fibrillation / Clinical Perspective. Circulation: Arrhythmia and Electrophysiology, 3 (1), 32-38. URL http://dx.doi.org/10.1161/CIRCEP.109.859116

[228] Health information privacy. United States Department of Health and Human Services. Retrieved August 01, 2011, from http://www.hhs.gov/ocr/privacy/

[229] Calkins, H., & Berger, R. 2011) Johns Hopkins special reports: atrial fibrillation: the latest management strategies. ePub.

[230] Paydek H. "Atrial Fibrillation After Radiofrequency Ablation of Type I Atrial Flutter," Circulation. 1998;98:p.315.

[231] Jais, P. Improved A-Fib Procedure. Summary of peer presentation. North American Society of Pacing and Electrophysiology Convention (NASPE), San Diego, CA May, 2002, San Diego. Retrieved July 31, 2011 from http://www.a-fib.com/HeartRhythmSociety2002.htm

[232] Haines, D. E. Atrial fibrillation: new approaches in management, presented by Dr. David Haines. (1999, August 10). [Transcript, Television broadcast]. University of Virginia School of Medicine. Retrieved July 31, 2011 from http://www.a-fib.com/HainesUnOfVirginiaAtrialFibrillation.htm

[233] Frost, L., Mølgaard, H., Christiansen, E. H., Hjortholm, K., Paulsen, P. K., & Thomsen, P. E. (1992). Atrial fibrillation and flutter after coronary artery bypass surgery: epidemiology, risk factors and preventive trials. International journal of cardiology, 36 (3), 253-261. Retrieved Aug. 5, 2011 from http://view.ncbi.nlm.nih.gov/pubmed/1358829

[234] Navarrete, A., Conte, F., Moran, M., Ali, I., & Milikan, N. (2011). Ablation of atrial fibrillation at the time of cavotricuspid isthmus ablation in patients with atrial flutter without documented atrial fibrillation derives a better Long-Term benefit. Journal of Cardiovascular Electrophysiology, 22 (1), 34-38. URL http://dx.doi.org/10.1111/j.1540-8167.2010.01845.x

[235] Chatterjee, S., Alexander, J. C., Pearson, P. J., & Feldman, T. (2011). Left atrial appendage occlusion: Lessons learned from surgical and transcatheter experiences. Ann Thorac Surg , 92 (6), 2283-2292. http://dx.doi.org/10.1016/j.athoracsur.2011.08.044

[236] Lubitz, S. A., Yin, X., Fontes, J. D. et al. (2010). Association between familial atrial fibrillation and risk of new-onset atrial fibrillation. JAMA. 304 (20), 2263-2269. URL http://dx.doi.org/10.1001/jama.2010.1690

[237] Brugada, R., Tapscott, T., Czernuszewicz, G. Z. et al. (1997). Identification of a genetic locus for familial atrial fibrillation. New England Journal of Medicine, 336 (13), 905-911. http://dx.doi.org/10.1056/NEJM199703273361302

[238] Ludwig-Maximilians-Universität München. (2010).When the heart gets out of step: Newly identified gene may open route to innovative treatments for atrial fibrillation Press release. Retrieved July 30, 2011 from http://www.eurekalert.org/pub_releases/2010-02/lm-wth021910.php

[239] Hughes, S. (2010, June 18). AtriClip for left atrial appendage occlusion approved in US. Theheart.org. Retrieved August 15, 2011, from http://www.theheart.org/article/1089215.do

[240] Daniel Doane: "When I relay what my doctors have told me, understand that I am paraphrasing from my probably inaccurate memory."

[241] Sutter Heart & Vascular Institute has been designated a Blue Distinction Center for Cardiac Care by Blue Cross. Sutter Memorial Video: TT Maze with recent patient story. Retrieved Aug. 5, 2011 from http://www.checksutterfirst.org/heartandvascular/videolibrary/ttmaze.html

[242] Longoria, J. (2010, July 22). Methods of treating a cardiac arrhythmia by thoracoscopic production of a Cox-Maze III lesion set. Patent application. PatentDocs. Retrieved Aug. 5, 2011 from http://www.faqs.org/patents/app/20100185186

[243] Longoria, J. and Wolff, L. Totally thoracoscopic epicardial RF ablation for atrial fibrillation using Atricure minimally invasive products. [Transcript, Television broadcast]. (2007, July 24). Sacramento, CA: ORLive.com. Retrieved August 5, 2011, from http://www.or-live.com/transcripts/2007/atr_1822_610.pdf

[244] Han, F. T., Kasirajan, V., Kowalski, M., et al. (2009). Results of a minimally invasive surgical pulmonary vein isolation and ganglionic plexi ablation for atrial fibrillation: single-center experience with 12-month follow-up. Circulation. Arrhythmia and electrophysiology, 2 (4), 370-377. URL http://dx.doi.org/10.1161/CIRCEP.109.854828

[245] Kron, J., Kasirajan, V., Wood, M. A., et al. (2010). Management of recurrent atrial arrhythmias after minimally invasive surgical pulmonary vein isolation and ganglionic plexi ablation for atrial fibrillation. Heart rhythm, 7 (4), 445-451. URL http://dx.doi.org/10.1016/j.hrthm.2009.12.008

[246] Marchlinski, F. Pulmonary Vein Isolation Alone for Long Standing Persistent A-Fib. Summary of peer presentation. Boston Atrial Fibrillation Symposium, Boston, MA. January, 14, 2011. Retrieved July 31, 2011 from http://www.a-fib.com/BostonA-FibSymposium2011.htm

[247] Wilber, D. (2011). Very late recurrence after catheter ablation of AF: Incidence and implications. Summary of peer presentation. Boston Atrial Fibrillation Symposium, Boston, MA. January, 14, 2011. Retrieved July 31, 2011 from http://www.a-fib.com/BostonA-FibSymposium2011.htm

[248] O'Riordan, M. (2011, January 5). Sobering long-term outcomes following ablation of atrial fibrillation. Theheart.org. Retrieved August 01, 2011, from http://www.theheart.org/article/1168671.do

[249] Sawhney, N., Anousheh, R., Chen, W.-C. C. et al. (2009). Five-year outcomes after segmental pulmonary vein isolation for paroxysmal atrial fibrillation. The American journal of cardiology, 104 (3), 366-372. URL http://dx.doi.org/10.1016/j.amjcard.2009.03.044

[250] Cohen, Todd J. A patient's guide to heart rhythm problems. Baltimore: Johns Hopkins UP, 2010. 36. Print.

[251] Radiofrequency catheter ablation is considered safe. (2010). AFIB Alliance: Atrial Fibrillation Resource. Retrieved August 01, 2011, from http://www.atrialfibrillation.com/medical-prof/therapy-outcome/safety

[252] Brown, M. T., & Bussell, J. K. (2011). Medication adherence: WHO cares? Mayo Clinic proceedings. Mayo Clinic , 86 (4), 304-314. URL http://dx.doi.org/10.4065/mcp.2010.0575

[253] Adán, V., & Crown, L. A. (2003). Diagnosis and treatment of sick sinus syndrome. American family physician, 67 (8), 1725-1732. Retrieved August 12, 2011, from http://view.ncbi.nlm.nih.gov/pubmed/12725451

[254] Medifocus guidebook on: atrial fibrillation: a comprehensive guide to symptoms, treatment, research, and support. Medifocus.com, Inc. July 2010. Vol. #CR004. 40. Print

[255] Rutherford David Rogers. American librarian: The New York Public Library (1954-1957); Library of Congress (1957-1964), Stanford University (1964-1969) and Yale University (1969-1985).

[256] Digital Object Identifier System. URL http://www.doi.org/index.html

Made in the USA
Coppell, TX
19 February 2023

13047843R10144